Caprice

My Boys My Body
My Business

BLINK

bringing you closer

Published by Blink Publishing
107-109 The Plaza,
535 King's Road,
Chelsea Harbour,
London, SW10 0SZ

www.blinkpublishing.co.uk

facebook.com/blinkpublishing
twitter.com/blinkpublishing

978-1-910536-03-2

Design by Blink Publishing

Printed and bound by Clays Ltd, St Ives Plc

1 3 5 7 9 10 8 6 4 2

Papers used by Blink Publishing are natural, recyclable products made from wood grown in sustainable forests. The manufacturing processes conform to the environmental regulations of the country of origin.

Blink Publishing is an imprint of the Bonnier Publishing Group
www.bonnierpublishing.co.uk

To my beautiful boys
You are my life
You are my happiness

Acknowledgements

'I am so excited to share my story with you. I hope it offers hope, inspiration – and puts a smile on your face.

I would like to thank my friends, family and gorgeous partner Ty for all their endless love, support and guidance.

Last but certainly not least, my boys!!

Jax and Jett, you fill my life with so much happiness and purpose. I love you with all of my heart and will try to be the best mommy I can and only hope as you grow older you will be as proud of Mommy as I am of you.'

Contents

Chapter 1

The Land of Opportunity

'What gorgeous thing am I going to wear today?' As my mom, Valerie, flung open her closet door I stood behind her, aghast at all the beautiful clothes she had to choose from.

Every morning my gorgeous, stylish, powerful mother would launch herself into the day with passion and enthusiasm and I loved and admired her for it. I wanted to emulate her, I wanted her to be proud of me and I wanted to create a life for myself at least as successful as the one she'd created for me.

It's fair to say that I am who I am because of my mom. As a single parent, she raised me to be as strong and go-getting as she was, and I owe my drive and my independent spirit to her.

'Cap,' she would declare with absolute certainty, 'happiness is independence. Never rely on anyone for anything – go out there and work hard and make your own money.'

I grew up with this sentiment drilled into me from the word go and so far, despite the rollercoaster ride my life has been, it's stood me in good stead.

I was not, contrary to what many people believe, raised on a trailer park with a car dealer for a dad. I was born on 24th October 1971 and raised in what used to be a very nice, middle-class area called Hacienda Heights, in California.

My mother, Valerie, was a stay-at-home mom at first. She didn't have to work because my father, Dale Bourret, ran his own business – Bourret Upholstery – and it was doing really well. We had plenty of money – and the trailer park story is pure bullshit.

I had an idyllic early childhood, even though my parents split up when I was four and I have no memory of my father living with us.

You know what? I have only two pictures of us as a family of four. Other than that, no 'happy family' shots, which is a little bit sad. But I know I loved my dad and he loved me, and he was my father. I continued to see him regularly for the few years after their split.

After the divorce, I was primarily raised without a dad because as the years went by, we saw less and less of him. It's certainly not a case of 'Oh, feel sorry for me, I come from a broken home'. It was just the way it was and, as I said, I am who I am because I was raised in a house with a very strong mother with a big personality.

Mom's big plan was to create her own interiors business and she knuckled down and worked her ass off creating Bourret Interiors, which still exists today and is doing very well. While she was setting up her business, my younger sister

Tiffany (forever called 'Tippy' by me) and I were growing up. It never occurred to us to really miss her, even though she was so busy and worked long hours, because we had Lupé, our housekeeper and nanny, an amazing but uber-strict Mexican lady, living with us from when I was a toddler until I was 16. Lupé ruled the house while Mom was at work.

Lupé was more than just our nanny; she was family. We loved her and she loved us. She was vibrant, warm and generous; I remember her buying me a pair of beautiful earrings in the shape of apples when I was a teenager. I was old enough then to realise that she had very little spare money so the fact that she was spending what she did have on me made those earrings even more precious.

But Lupé was tough too! She'd scream at us when we were naughty and if we ignored her, we were in the dog-house. And, boy, could she be a drama queen. At least twice a year, we'd have to call an ambulance because Lupé was convinced she was dying: 'I'm having a heart attack, I'm really having a heart attack!' she would say, coming hysterically into the living room in a panic, her face bright red and sweating. Each time we were so frightened we'd call 911 and each time it turned out just to be heartburn, because Lupé ate the hottest chillies ever! She was an amazing cook, and gave me a lifelong love of Mexican food. I could have jalapeño peppers with everything.

My mom's family all lived close by and so we had lots of support. Most of them were within ten minutes of the house and so if Lupé or Mom weren't around, my grandma and nana would take my sister and me to school, and we spent a lot of time with them over the years.

Our family home was full-on seventies-a-rama. We had garish wallpaper, orange curtains, that dark-green swirly carpet, smoked glass coffee tables – the whole nine yards. My mom was making a lot of money and we had all the latest gadgets and we wore nice clothes, but we certainly weren't spoiled. 'I want my girls to have the best of everything!' she'd declare, and because my mother is a force of nature, she'd make it happen.

We had a pretty idyllic childhood in a warm, happy household with lots of pets – especially dogs. My earliest memory still filters into my dreams, even now. We always had dogs and I can remember seeing our pet collie, Rusty, as he stared at me through a glass patio door. He kept gazing at me, it was if it was right into my soul (well, that's what it felt like). I looked back at him and I just knew in my heart there was something wrong. I remember giving him a big hug and soon after, my mom took him away to the vets and came back later without him.

How I howled with grief. I can't have been more than eight years old but that memory has stayed with me ever since. It was really traumatising. Animals were a big part of our family life: I learned to ride when I was tiny and when my mom bought a holiday home in Hawaii my sister and I would ride across the fabulous beaches there. I have amazing memories of that time.

Family was everything to me. We weren't religious in any major way. We didn't go to synagogue or celebrate any of the big Jewish high days or holidays like Hanukkah, at least not until I was a teenager.

Friday night dinner was the traditional time for my family

to get together. A feast was prepared, and the entire family would descend on us – aunts, uncles, grandparents. There were about 20 of us digging into a delicious meal every Friday.

But we had a little twist on the convention. Once we'd devoured the food, someone would yell: 'It's poker time!' and that would be it – the cards would be out and we'd still be playing at 2am. The whole family, no matter what age, would play. Not for money, just for plastic chips. That is how I learned to be a poker expert at the tender age of 13 – a strategic skill that was to come in very useful later on in my life.

Our Friday night dinners also gave me an innate love of family and I absolutely adore the chaos of having my kids and step-kids around me. Bring it on! Bring your friends! It's such a wonderful, warm feeling having people who care for each other all together.

You'd think that with all this family surrounding me, I'd have been a confident, gregarious child – especially in light of the life I've gone on to lead. But in fact I was very shy, very sweet and innocent, and I wouldn't say boo to a goose. Tippy was a lot more feisty, but we were pretty much joined at the hip because we were so close in age. Tippy looked – still looks – exactly like mom. I don't look like my mom or my dad. Seriously, I could come from the milkman! The only person I look remotely like is my dad's mom, Grandma Doris, who died in 1987 when I was 15.

Tippy was most definitely the rebel of the family. She has the biggest personality and she's really witty and effortlessly smart. I had to work very hard for my As in high school; Tippy, on the other hand, seemed to get them without much effort.

I remember once, when I was about eight years old and Tippy was six, she got really mad at me. She came charging at me with a kitchen knife she'd grabbed out of the drawer screaming she was going to kill me! Lupé said: '*Ay chi wawa Estafani, ay chi wawa!*' (which was her exclamation for: 'What the hell are you doing?' I guess and she always called Tippy 'Estafani'). Thankfully, disaster was always averted but we'd be forever fighting in that natural, sibling way.

Remember that Van Halen song, 'Jump'? Tippy would play that in front of the whole family on a Friday night, put golf balls up her jumper and pretend she had boobies. She'd play air guitar and sing along to this massive rock anthem. She was so theatrical that Mom was convinced she'd go into acting or performing of some sort but in fact when she was older Tippy just wanted the stability of a solid family. Tippy's life these days couldn't be more removed from those childhood theatrics: she now works with very sick children. I have huge respect for my sister; it's a very tough, selfless job she does.

The first few years after my parents' divorce, I saw a lot of my dad, who'd remarried a lady who had two girls of her own. The girls were the same age as Tippy and I and actually we all got on really well. It was a great time for me. At the weekends we'd disappear off up to Dad's home. He had a beautiful house not far from ours in an area called La Habra Heights, with horses and a pool.

While my mom was busy creating this amazing life for us, she was having a pretty good social life of her own! My mom was a hottie (still is, in case you're reading this, Mom!) and she had hundreds of boyfriends. Not that she brought them home – we rarely met any of them – but we just somehow got it: the guys liked Mom and she liked them, nothing at all wrong with that. Except that sometimes her admirers weren't the kind she wanted.

I shudder to think of it now but one episode will stay with me forever.

I was taking a shower one night in my mom's en suite bathroom, when I was maybe ten or eleven years old. I suddenly had that prickly feeling you get when you just know someone's looking at you. I glanced out from behind the shower door – luckily it was frosted glass – to see a swarthy-looking guy staring at me and then looking down at my mom's jewellery that was spread out across her dressing table.

I was absolutely paralysed with fear. He was dressed in brown overalls with short sleeves, almost like prison garb.

Did he want to hurt me, or even worse? Oh my god, I was wet, naked and just two feet in front of him. That's ridiculous, I thought, why would anyone want a teenager with seven pubic hairs and bee stings for boobies? Before I knew it, he ran out of the bathroom without hurting me or stealing any of Mom's diamonds. I was safe. I grabbed a towel and ran into the living room. Mom was glued to the TV, watching *Dallas*. 'Mom, that was the worst so-called joke you've ever played on me. Are you sick? What's wrong with you?' I thought she'd persuaded one of my uncle's friends to pretend like he was a stalker, just to see how I'd react.

'What are you talking about?' she exclaimed. I told her what had happened and I could see the fear and panic in her eyes. She called the police instantly. Twenty minutes later, three police cars arrived. They were with us for about

90 minutes, then we all walked outside to escort the police to their cars and thank them for their time.

The next thing we knew, a man in brown overalls was running for his life up the side of our hill, right next to the cop cars. He had been hiding behind our brick wall for the whole time. I screamed hysterically: 'That's him, that's him!' The police went running after him but they never caught him.

It turns out he was on the Most Wanted list in Orange County and was referred to as the Orange County Rapist. He'd savagely raped several ladies over the past year. When my mom found out about this she put bars on all the windows and doors – it was like living in Fort Knox but we felt safe. We were very fortunate to have escaped this monster.

Events as menacing as this were one-offs. My mother is a strong lady, but even so, it's hard not to feel vulnerable as a woman living alone with two young daughters, no matter how tough you think you are. Mom did have a long-term boyfriend, a really lovely guy called Latif who was Kuwaiti. She was with him for around eight years and he was a wonderful step-dad. He was great fun and we adored him.

Latif went back to Kuwait during the Gulf War when Saddam Hussein's forces occupied the country in 1990, and tragically he was killed. My mom was devastated. I have very happy memories of him and my mom together.

It was around this time that my mom decided to take my dad to court because my dad had stopped paying for child support, school fees and medical fees. He just stopped paying altogether. She won the case and the judge awarded my mom child support and back-payment of $45,000 – but my dad just never paid it.

He was a well-to-do man living in one of the best neighbourhoods in our area. He had horses and a swimming pool, and he was refurbing his mansion. His step-daughters, who were the same age as Tippy and me, were both at private schools and he had a thriving business. He was very, very wealthy. I just don't know why a father wouldn't want to support his kids – it wasn't a lot of money to him. Why did he get himself into so much debt with the child maintenance? My mom wasn't awarded a huge amount in the first place because she was successful in her own right and so I don't know why he stopped paying and refused to pay even when ordered to by the court. In the end, my mom couldn't stand it any more and she just dropped the claim.

My mom had come to a realisation that she was never going to get the money she was owed and she couldn't keep going back to court. She had to just let it go and move on. Instead, she had a new-found hunger to make money as she was on her own and she wanted to give Tippy and me the best upbringing possible. It's not easy being a single mom with no financial support and my mom worked very hard to give us a good life.

We had a beautiful holiday home in Hawaii, we had a nanny, we went to private schools – we even had an award-winning race-horse at one point called Big City Miss.

In the end, regardless of the judgement, my dad didn't pay one cent to my mom, and by the time I was 9 years old Tippy and I were no longer seeing my dad. We just stopped going. He stopped asking us to go. It became too difficult. I'm sure if I ever do manage to talk this through with him, Dad would have good reasons why he no longer saw us. To be fair, there are always two sides to every story and I'm sure he has some valid reason why… Or at least, I like to think so.

The acrimony between Mom and Dad affected my sister and me in different ways. Where as Tippy settled down quickly, it put me permanently off marriage. I mean, you come together as two people, you have a family together and it ends like this? The damage it does to the children and their future, it's just not worth it. I am really not interested and it's the reason I didn't commit to any relationship for a very long time. I was all about the fun and if it stopped being fun, I moved on.

I hate the way marriage becomes about money in this way. I understand that if you give up your career to have kids and be a full-time mom, then you need financial support if your marriage breaks up, but if you have enough money to look after yourself and your kids, putting yourself through a depressing legal battle seems like such an unnecessary evil. Why not do a 'pinky swear' and say, 'I love you, let's try and make this work for the rest of our lives, and if we're making each other miserable we'll go our separate ways.' It's so toxic when money gets involved.

I don't think that growing up without a dad throughout my teenage years affected me as much as it might other people. I had such a strong role model in my mom and so much family around me, it made little difference. I saw so much of my male cousins and my uncles, and they were my father figures. And I was a teenager! I was busy with my friends and my school life and my weekends were filled with going to the mall and socialising. I just got on with my life.

As time has gone on, I guess I realise Dad did the best he

could. I think to dwell on why we lost touch is just damaging psychologically. I'd rather be in this bubble I'm in where I'm happy with the way I feel towards him. Besides, I owe certain attributes of my personality to him: he's a kind man who really wants to believe the best in people; if someone does something wrong, he'll always be the one saying, 'They're a good person, they'll figure it out,' and he won't make a big deal of it.

The one person I was adamant I couldn't lose touch with though, was my wonderful Grandma Doris, my dad's mom. I thought she was the kindest, most beautiful woman I'd ever met and I loved spending time with her.

Grandma Doris was achingly elegant, cultured and generous to a fault, with everyone. She didn't live far from us and even after the divorce, she continued to get on well with Mom and would come and see us at the house – always with gifts. Mom would drop us off at Grandma's house regularly too, and Tippy and I loved that. I can still smell the divine French toast she would make for us – it remains the best I've ever tasted.

Grandma was such a significant person in my life that when she got diagnosed with pancreatic cancer when I was 16, I was utterly devastated. I couldn't accept that she was going to die; how could she? She was a huge part of my life and it hurt just to think she might not be there forever.

During that period, I remember visiting Grandma at her house and the strange, sickly smell of her illness permeating through every room. Watching her deteriorate was truly awful. This lively, interesting, gentle, fun lady was a shell of her former self.

The day Grandma died my mother took the call from Dad's sister, Diana. My auntie broke the news to Tippy and I and I remember doubling over with distress. How could my precious grandma have passed? I needed her. I couldn't imagine life without her.

To make a sad situation much, much worse, Auntie Diana refused to let my sister and me attend the funeral. The relationship between my parents must have reached such depths that they wanted no more to do with any of us. Even now, this makes me so sad. I wish it could have been different.

Tippy and I defied them though. Nothing was going to stop us paying our respects to our beloved Grandma Doris. So we went to the funeral, even though we knew we weren't wanted. We sat at the back of the church away from the rest of the family and afterwards no one comforted the two teenage girls sobbing outside the church. I cannot imagine what was going through their minds and to this day I will not talk to Auntie Diana.

Years later, Diana visited England and tried to get in touch to see if she could stay at my house, but I didn't respond. I was still really hurt about the way my sister and I were treated at my grandma's funeral.

I also remember another incident at school around this time, when I was in seventh grade and started being bullied by an eighth grader. A girl called Jodie – an 'indie' kid at my school – just loved intimidating me. I'd feel her eyes boring into me in the schoolyard or the cafeteria.

'What you looking at?' she'd demand, even when my eyes were firmly glued to the floor. It never escalated into a fight but she kept harassing me all throughout the year. I couldn't stand going to school as a result.

She was a pretty girl herself, but I guess being one of the 'alternative' crowd, she liked to intimidate sweet little innocent girls who wouldn't hurt a fly; she felt empowered by that. Maybe there was something going on at home and that's why she became a bully but, whatever, she knew I would never dream of standing up to her.

But eighth grade? I loved it. That year I got into the cheerleading team and in order to do that, I had to make up my own cheer, which was a bit nerve-racking at the time because I'd never done anything like it before. I still remember my try-out cheer to this day and I'm going to share it with you but please don't judge me!

We're heading for success,
passing by all the rest,
S.U.C.C.E.S.S. we are the best!

Later on that year I actually became one of the team captains of the cheerleaders and, although I was still very shy, my confidence began to grow.

When I was 13, I sat the entrance exams for two private high schools. My mom would have to pay astronomical fees to send us, but she wanted the very best for my sister and me. I passed both exams but we chose Bishop Amat, a very exclusive private school nearby, and my sister followed me there two years later.

I absolutely loved the early years at Bishop Amat. During my sophomore year (this is the second year of high school) I was one of the captains of the cheerleading squad and also homecoming queen. Being homecoming queen or King is a huge deal in the States. The voting is done in secret and other students vote for the person they feel has contributed most to the life of the school. It's really prestigious and so, of course, I was beyond thrilled to win.

I'd been on the Honour Roll (the students who do well in all their subjects make up this list) for the year as well as taking part in all kinds of sports. I guess it all counted in the votes.

I had plenty of friends to begin with at Bishop Amat, and I just enjoyed hanging out with them and being a regular kid. Yes, I did enter beauty pageants (which I hated) but despite what you might think, they didn't give me a big ego (believe me, that would come much later!). I was still a really normal, innocent kid, going to the mall with my friends, flirting with boys (but not taking it anywhere), and seeing a lot of my family.

Like most of my friends, I was heavily into the music of the era, and posters of bands such as The Smiths and Depeche Mode were all over my bedroom walls. I had a big crush on Dave Gahan from Depeche Mode, and even now, I know I'd revert back to that star-struck 15-year-old if I should happen to meet him. I loved all the British indie music – though I didn't feel quite the same about Morrissey as I did about Dave.

My mom was happy because all my friends were nice,

privately educated kids from good backgrounds. That didn't mean that they all had charmed lives, and there is one horrific incident relating to a really good friend of mine, that I'll never forget.

One night, about 4am, this friend called me, utterly hysterical. 'Cap, you have to come, you've gotta come over,' she was babbling, practically incoherent. She got me really worried. I was old enough to drive by this time so I talked to my mom straight away and said, 'Look, I don't know what's wrong but I need to go over.'

What I saw when I arrived at her house will never leave me. My friend's five-year-old brother had found their mom hanging in the garage, with a chain deeply embedded around her neck. The poor child was in shock and my friend was sobbing hysterically. I went into shock myself. When I arrived at her front door the body was there and you could see the chain marks around her neck. This was the first and hopefully the last time I will ever see a dead body. In the middle of our comfortable, middle-class existence someone had chosen to take their own life in such a horrific way.

After the suicide was investigated it emerged that her mom was part of some kind of cult, but what caused her to get involved with such a cult, and ultimately do something so awful, we'll never know. Up until this point, her mom had always seemed to us to be a normal, nurturing loving person, and this made the shock even greater. I haven't seen my friend for many years but I think of her often and I really hope she's managed to come to terms with what happened that night.

It was a deeply upsetting and traumatic event but something so beyond 'normal' life that the only way we could all deal with it was to be there for our friend, focus on high school and get on with day-to-day living.

By the time my senior year came around, my friends were dropping off the radar. If you ask my mom, she insists other girls were jealous and I was ostracised, because I was doing well at my studies and winning pageants. Mom would say: 'It's all because my daughter was the most beautiful girl in school.' She was biased, obviously, all moms are! But I think people did have the idea that I was Princess Perfect, and that view was only backed up when I dated the captain of the football team of an opposing school. That's pretty much hitting the jackpot in Highschoolville. Whatever it was down to, it must have faded, because I was voted Prom Queen that year.

I got my first boyfriend (the captain of the football team) when I was 15, and we went out for just a few months. It was all very innocent and I was still a virgin when we split up. It wasn't until later, when I won Miss Teen California, that I met my first 'proper' boyfriend, Tor.

I was 17 and Tor was two years older than me. What a name, right? Well he looked like a Viking god, too, I can tell you!

Tor was attending the Miss Teen California competition and when I won, he made a beeline for me! Why did I fall for him? Because he was stunningly gorgeous! He was the hottest guy I'd ever seen. I have to admit, looks really mattered to me back then – and still do. OK, I'm little bit superficial but nobody's perfect, right?

We ended up going out for three years, until I moved to New York to work as a model. Not only did he look divine, he was also a Chippendale dancer. So there I was, Miss Teen California, driving around in a fabulous Fiero sports car bought for me by my mom, with my Chippendale dancer beside me. I thought I was the bees' knees!

Tor was a lovely guy. I adored him – and so did my mom. I couldn't wait to go to my high school prom, the most important night of the school calendar, with him on my arm. It was also the night I was crowned Prom Queen, so the expectations for the evening were pretty high.

Unfortunately, this sparkling evening didn't turn out quite as expected. It had a magical start, when Tor turned up at my house in his dinner suit looking completely adorable, ready to escort me to my special night. But just as Tor and I hit the dance floor, dressed to the nines and looking eighties-fabulous, a couple of kids suddenly tore towards us. 'It's Tippy! She's convulsing!' they yelled, and dragged me off to see my sister.

Tippy had been invited by a guy in my year called Kristian and she had been pretty thrilled to be on the arm of a senior. But by the time I reached her in the bathroom, poor Tippy was lying on the floor, convulsing horribly. I don't know to this day what caused it in the bathroom. Tests didn't show up anything and it's never happened since, thankfully. But when the ambulance turned up and we were whisked off to the hospital, I spent my prom night out of my mind with worry for my sister…

Considering that as a teenager I must have looked like the perfect all-American homecoming queen/cheerleader/ Miss Goodie-Two-Shoes (which I kind of was), deep down I still didn't have much confidence, and some of my good friends had dropped away by the time I reached my last year at high school.

When I was around 14 years old, my mom decided it was pageant time. This was not – I repeat, *not* – something I wanted to do. I blame my mom! Mind you, she wasn't the only one. Lots of the parents were really into entering their kids in beauty pageants. It was part of the culture at that time. These events were the highlights of their year! I loved my mom so much I'd have done anything to make her happy.

Tippy escaped the whole crazy experience because my mom just knew she wouldn't do it. Tippy was always the one who would backtalk my mom and refuse point-blank to do something if she didn't want to. Stubborn, headstrong, dramatic… just like mom! When it came to pageants? Forget it!

It wasn't a question of favouritism – me getting to do the pageants and ignoring Tip – no, it was because I was left to do all the fluffy bullshit!

Meanwhile, my mom and I would traipse from one contest to another and those pageants required lots of preparation and a hell of a lot of money to pull off. You know that movie, *Miss Congeniality*? The bitchiness and the dirty deeds are not exaggerated. In fact they have nothing on what goes on behind the scenes at real beauty pageants!

It wasn't uncommon for dresses to be stolen. I'll never forget the day one of my dresses went missing. 'My dress has gone!' I screamed. It was like the end of the world. In the scramble to get ready, my tailor-made evening gown, which had taken weeks to make and had cost around $800, had disappeared. Taken by a jealous rival. Yes! This stuff really happens. Any time anyone felt you were a threat to the crown, you were in danger, and I guess that's why the competitors never really became friends with me. It just wasn't going to happen in that kind of atmosphere.

Those pageants must have cost my mom thousands upon thousands over the years. We usually had to have a bathing suit, an evening gown and then another set of clothes for the interviews and the shows. It was insane the amount of time and effort it took up – and I was a girl who hated wearing make-up!

Did it give me a taste for the limelight? No! I couldn't stand pageants! At that time I wasn't interested in anything other than politics (yes, really. I'll explain in a minute.) or becoming a high-powered businesswoman like Leona Helmsley. Helmsley, at that time, had built herself up as an entrepreneur in the hotel business and was a huge name in the States for being this ball-breaker of a businesswoman.

Unfortunately, she was later indicted for tax evasion and spent 19 months in jail, at which point she ceased to be my role model! But when I was younger, Leona encapsulated all I aspired to: independent wealth and strength of character. Just like my mom, in fact. It's interesting that my role models were always female. From around the age of eight, I began to have this burning ambition and my mom recognised that about me and encouraged it. I guess the least I could do was go along with the beauty pageants!

At this point, as a 14-year-old, I developed a big interest in politics, believe it or not. I was obsessed and I'd read books constantly about the US political system and the big players involved. It wasn't anything to do with homework, I did it all off my own back.

I guess from that interest, I began volunteering for various charities. I volunteered at a hospital that looked after mentally handicapped people. And I'd go there on my own after school for a good few years. It was hard work but very humbling for me. It gave me an understanding of just how hard some people's lives are and that's really stayed with me. In some way, I must have realised just how lucky I was and that sense of wanting to give something back has never left me.

As soon as I went into modelling, even when I had very little money, I'd still send off my $10 off every month to World Vision – a charity that helps children in poverty. It wasn't much, but I had so little of my own money, it seemed a lot at the time.

So alongside this wonderful world of pageantry, I was developing some sort of social conscience. Looking back, maybe one balanced out the other – I certainly hoped that one day I'd be able to use money or influence to help other people and it's something I still feel strongly about to this day.

Mom didn't just hand money to us willy-nilly. She expected me to get a job and I wanted to earn my own money anyway. I was 17 and still in high school when I found work in a women's boutique called Red Eye and it was my job to help ladies choose clothes and try them on.

My style was definitely not to be all over customers as they walked in the shop. People don't like it. I hated being bothered by shop assistants then and I hate it now. I remember trying to tell the manager of the store, 'I don't think this is a good tactic, I think it scares people away!' and I got fired after about a month!

After the boutique job, I found work at a very posh restaurant called Top of the Brea. I was the hostess with the mostest in the restaurant. I had to show people to their seats and I earned peanuts for it. I remember one Valentine's Day and a guy turned up on his first date with a girl and even though there was at least a two-hour wait, I managed to find them a secluded corner table immediately. He was so grateful he gave me a $5 tip. I was so excited I almost lost the plot! I'd never been tipped that much money before. Usually I wouldn't make that kind of money in two hours. I'm so glad I worked these jobs because they taught me early on about customer service and looking after people.

Everything changed for me in 1989 when I won Miss Teen California, and my world kind of tipped on its axis.

I was on a total high after winning the pageant. This was a big one and I couldn't believe I'd won. If you look at the photographs taken at the event, you can see me in tears. It was all very dramatic! A smartly dressed woman approached me as I emerged from the backstage area into a seething mob of people wanting to congratulate me and take pictures. They were even asking for autographs. I couldn't believe what was happening to me.

And then, out of the throng, the woman approached me with a broad smile and her business card. 'I'd like to sign you up, I think you could make a lot of money as a model.' Was this my chance? I had never considered making a living out of modelling – the pageants had just been a hobby to please Mom and, as I said, I was more interested in going into politics or business. But at this moment, a light bulb went on in my head.

It dawned on me that unexpectedly I had the opportunity to forge a future for myself as a model and make real money. And who knows where it might lead? It looked like the American Dream was mine for the taking.

When I look back over that time, it seems fate was intervening to force me to grow up, and fast. Within months of me winning Miss Teen California, my grandfather, Mom's dad, passed away, also of pancreatic cancer. Within a year I had lost Grandma Doris and my mom's own father to the same brutal disease. I have a very clear memory of sitting outside my grandfather's house and my uncle coming to tell us he'd passed, and from that moment on, our lives were to change.

My mom was incredibly close to her father, and she spoke to him every day without fail; he was her sunshine. When he died, Mom fell to pieces. It was heart-wrenching to watch this dynamic, powerful, amazing woman deteriorate in front of my eyes. It was as if her dad dying just blew all the fight out of her.

My mom went from having a really successful business, travelling, playing racketball for two hours every day and with great friends, to stopping everything overnight. She didn't want to talk to anyone, she didn't want help from anyone; she was in a very bad way.

Over the next few years Mom would lose everything – and I mean everything – because she just couldn't function. She was declared bankrupt, we lost my childhood home and that was it for almost the next ten years of her life. She just crashed and burned.

She says now she doesn't remember too much from that time. Thankfully life now has completely turned around for her and I suppose that's why she's able to be so open about this period in her life. It has made her stronger and wiser. When she bounced back, Bourret Interiors bounced back to net seven figures, and Mom would eventually buy a gorgeous building to work out of. Not just an office... the whole damn building! She is an inspiration, and she certainly made me aware of how fragile success can be.

I was on the brink of flying the nest to make my own way in the world and Mom told me to go. 'Get out there and make some money,' were her words. She couldn't look after me; she was having too tough a time of her own.

Years later, I fell into a similar state and Mom helped prevent my depression from turning into something long-term. She wasn't particularly sympathetic towards me but maybe her toughness was her absolute fear of my condition spiralling the way hers did.

I did manage a semester at college – studying ppolitical science – but by this point my new modelling career was starting to show promise and because I had a way out, a way to carve a future away from the sadness at home, I took it. I closed the door on my childhood home for the last time and took the big step of moving to LA.

It was the spring of 1990 and this was my first ever shoot – for a calendar, very glam. I remember being flown out to a tropical paradise and posing in gorgeous, expensive, designer swimsuits. Inside, I was hugging myself with excitement. I was actually getting paid, for a job I wanted to do, with prospects!

'OK, Caprice, give me a big smile, I want you to look straight into the camera and make this picture come alive!'

The photographer seemed pleased with the way I was posing. 'You're a pro already!' he grinned at me. 'You certainly have great presence in front of the camera'. It was to be the first of a series of pretty straightforward jobs I did for catalogues but it was incredibly exciting to me – and I was getting money for it!

I moved into a tiny apartment in Hollywood with my friend Susie, who'd I'd been at junior high with. Don't get the wrong impression though: Hollywood glamour it was not, but it was our first experience of independence and we loved it. I did have a waterbed though! It was the nineties, of course I had a waterbed – it was the bollocks! I brought it with me from my home in Hacienda Heights. There was no way I was leaving that baby behind for someone else to enjoy!

Susie was modelling too and we'd go to castings together, shop together and just have fun partying, but we had very little spare money once we'd paid the rent. My sister was still living at home with Mom and I'd keep in constant touch with her and go home at weekends to see them. Mom wasn't in a good way. Family members rallied around but it was difficult for her. She's such a proud person and she wouldn't accept help; little did we know then how long her recovery would be.

In the meantime, I made friends with a girl called Barbara Baldieri who is still one of my dearest friends in the world.

The two of us would end up on the same photo shoots all the time, often doing catalogues of one sort or another, and an occasional calendar. She was the brunette, I was the blonde and it became a bit of a joke. We were booked for every single job together, we were the same age and we were both just starting out. Great times… but after about eighteen months, fate was about to intervene once more.

As with a lot of model agencies, then and now, the bigger New York agencies were always looking out for new talent, and a lady called Victoria had seen my model card – these are A5 sized cards covered with your best photos and in the days before the internet, they'd be sent to prospective clients before they called you in for a casting. At the time it was the rise of Kate Moss. Glam was out and models with an interesting and unique look were in. But there was still a massive market for wholesome-looking sexy blondes and I guess I fitted that bill. One day, as I was sat there painting my nails at home, I got a call out of the blue.

'Hi Caprice, this is Victoria.' Victoria was the modelling booker who started everything for me. She thought I needed to go to New York because that is where the big money is made as a model. Big-money modelling? I kind of assumed I was already making pretty good money.

But I was listening, because this lady clearly meant business. Victoria offered to pay for my flight and sort out my accommodation and told me she'd meet me at the airport… I realised she wasn't pushy, just professional. My instincts told me she was a good person to know and I was proved right. 'OK, I'll be there!' I said, sounding as confident as possible – feeling like jelly inside!

This time, despite my nerves, there was no doubt in my mind, I had to go to the Big Apple – it both scared and excited me. It did mean leaving behind my mom and sister as well as Susie and Barbara but of course, at that time I had no idea I'd be leaving California for good…

Chapter 2

The Dream Takes Flight

I approached LAX airport with my heart in my mouth. This was really it. If everything can change on the throw of a dice, this was my moment at the gaming table.

It was 28th August 1993 and it was a day of firsts – first time on a plane alone, first time I'd been such a distance from my mom and sister and certainly the first time I was landing in a city where I knew no one. It was exciting, exhilarating – and terrifying! As I sat on the five-hour flight between LA and New York I could hardly bear to sit still.

What if Victoria changed her mind when she saw me and thought I'd never make it big-time as a model after all? Or what if she was wrong and I couldn't get any work? How would I pay my rent when I had no back-up (my mom had lost everything by this point and I would never ask my dad for money)? So many questions ran through my mind. So many anxieties.

It really was like jumping off a cliff and hoping beyond hope there was a trampoline waiting for me at the bottom to bounce me back up again.

But then, as I looked out at the great big city that I was leaving behind sprawling beneath the airplane, I allowed myself a wriggle of excitement. This was my big chance and I must not blow it.

Victoria, true to her word, was waiting for me at JFK airport, a few miles out of New York City. As we sat in the taxi into town, I felt suddenly shy. It all looked so overwhelming as we came over the bridge and I glimpsed the iconic cityscape of Manhattan. I was just 19 years old. Who was I to think I could make something of a career here? It was a moment of self-doubt but Victoria must have sensed it because she was soon talking nineteen-to-the-dozen about her plans for me. My relief must have been palpable. Victoria was a great mentor to me then, and a big part of my journey to success. She's brilliant, and we are still in touch.

Half an hour later Victoria was showing me into an apartment in the Worldwide Plaza on West 50th Street. It was a really rough area at the time and though I was going to be living in a penthouse apartment, the rent was very cheap. The only furniture was a bed – but the view was great and it could have been the Four Seasons hotel as far as I was concerned. It felt like I'd truly arrived.

My rent for the apartment came out of my earnings and in those early days it wasn't always easy to make it but somehow I scraped together enough each month to get through. It was hard at times.

I was still basically a kid, and I could barely afford to feed myself. I lived on pad thai – that filling Thai noodle dish – and bagels, for months and months. I was so skinny! Not because I'd been told to lose weight for the job, just because I had no money to buy food!

During the first few months I spent most of my time getting to know the streets of New York by traipsing from one casting to the next. My boyfriend Tor and I split up after I arrived in the city because I think, really, he wanted marriage and babies. He'd been such an important person in my life but after what I'd seen my parents go through there was no way I was going down that road... and so the relationship was doomed. I don't know where he is now but he was such a sweet guy, I'm sure he's made someone a wonderful husband and father.

Yes, I missed home badly at times, but I couldn't afford to fly back to see my family. I knew Mom was in a bad way, from conversations with her and Tippy, and this made it very, very hard. That first winter, freezing my ass off as I went around the city in the snow, touting for work, was often pretty bleak, and I spent a lot of my time off shivering in that apartment with a bare food cupboard. I often wondered if I should just haul my ass back to sunny LA.

The agency had taken me on because I had this kind of all-American wholesome-but-sexy thing going on and I had a butt and I had curves and, as I've said, this kind of look was the opposite of the 'heroin chic' vibe that so many of the fashion crowd loved at that time. I'm not knocking the likes of Kate Moss, not at all, she's incredible. But I'm thankful there was, and still is, room for different looks and body types in the fashion world, just like there is in life in general!

It was during this period that the supermodels were big business. They were quite aloof and I got the feeling that they looked down on us girls who were just starting out. Stephanie Seymour was nice though as was Carla Bruni but generally, the Supers were on a different planet from the rest of us.

So, yeah, my first year was really tough, but it didn't mean I wasn't enjoying myself. I was so lucky. I was young, free and single and having the time of my life (apart from feeling hungry all the time, living off those bagels). And New York was a hotbed of fun parties, though I didn't drink in those days because I needed to keep my head together and I was scared of losing control. I was to stay that way for another ten years.

There were a lot of drugs around, though not the kind of drugs you read about today – ketamine and crack – it was more common for people to use coke, Quaaludes and magic mushrooms. Me? I've tried drugs twice and it was enough to put me off forever.

One cold winter's night in the city we were round at some guy's house – let's call him John. He was probably around 23, I was still only 19, and we were partying with some other models and his friends, one of whom suggested I try the mushrooms.

Naively, I just wanted to fit in, I didn't want to be a goober. So I ate a couple of these revolting-tasting dried mushrooms. I'd obviously not done enough research because I know now they can take a while to kick in and you need to wait for this to happen before deciding, as I did, that the mushrooms aren't having any hallucinatory effect whatsoever and you need to take more.

I was curious, I wanted to know what mind-expanding events would occur, if I learn more about myself. Would I see beautiful things about the world I'd never seen before? Maybe the Californian in me wanted to see the glorious, vibrant colours of my home territory in a corner of New York. Whatever. Unfortunately, this is not what happened.

I had what's known as a bad trip. It started out OK. A few of us went outside into the snow to watch a light show that was on nearby. I then started to laugh hysterically, I was literally crying with laughter as the man to the right of me morphed into this big green frog. He looked exactly like Kermit from the Muppets.

My friends quickly took me back to John's apartment. I went snooping around and found myself in his room. He had a gorgeous balcony on the 67th floor overlooking the city. I was convinced I could fly from his balcony to the adjacent roof of the next building. I was really excited about this new super-power I had. So I proceeded to climb the glass rail… Thankfully, John burst into the room screaming, 'Don't jump!' at me and grabbed me and slammed me to the floor.

He locked me in the bathroom and at that point I was acting a little irrationally. I rolled up into a tight ball and prayed all through the night as I felt there was a dark force after me. I think I prayed for about seven hours straight until finally the light came back into my life again and I fell into an exhausted sleep. When I woke up that afternoon on the floor of the bathroom there was blood all over my face, my hands and my arms. I had eaten up the insides of my cheek; I must have been chewing and chewing all night long as I couldn't speak or chew for days because I'd been grinding my teeth so persistently.

It was a horrible experience, but you know what? It was a blessing in disguise, because it put me off taking any drugs again. Later on, I'd regularly be in situations where drugs were available, but that first time was my last (at least by choice – but more of that later). I'm not interested in doing any drugs – not even a joint.

I spent two years in New York and that second year, things really began to take off for me. Hey, I could even afford a sofa for the apartment! I finally moved on from the dreaded pad thai and bagel diet. This change was all down to me landing my first ever magazine cover: *Vogue Mexico* – thanks to my agent Victoria, who hyped me up and got me the booking. It was a real game changer for me.

Up until that point, the kind of work I was getting was pretty varied: I'd do some catwalk and some calendar work but I never really cracked the high fashion market because I was a traditional looking, pretty girl rather than an uber-skinny coat-hanger of a model, which is what's usually needed for the haute couture side of the market.

Landing a *Vogue* cover definitely elevates a model to a whole new level. Designers take you more seriously, and you're much more likely to get auditions for major designer castings. Even then, the nearest I got to a major designer casting me was from a 'go-see' with the legend that is Ralph Lauren. All Ralph's girls look like wholesome thoroughbreds. I guess I slotted into this role – or hoped I did.

With some trepidation, I went to his studio to meet Mr Lauren, who was busy seeing girl after girl. I gave him my sweetest smile, he considered me from all angles and then to my horror I remembered I'd left my red nail polish on my toes.

'What's the big deal', you might ask. But with all model castings you're supposed to turn up 'clean'. Clean hair and absolutely no make-up on your face. I'd made sure of that and I looked as scrubbed and wholesome as can be. But then his eyes dropped to my toes (I was wearing open-toed sandals) and that was it – 'Next,' he said in a clipped, slightly irritated voice. And just like that, I'd blown my one and only Ralph Lauren casting because of the shiny red nail polish on my toenails. I knew I'd never get that chance again!

But one door closes and another one opens, and I did land a lingerie campaign with Calvin Klein, which was my second big job after *Vogue*, and what really started to get me noticed. I was also on the cover of another magazine called *Accessories*, which was quite a coup at the time. Bookings started to come in but I still didn't have enough variety in my 'book' – my portfolio – to secure the designer work and to bring in some of the bigger contracts with major brands.

Victoria called me in to see her one day and said: 'Listen, Cap, we gotta get you some more tear-sheets so you can win the big campaigns.' What she meant was that I needed to do more creative fashion photo shoots with different photographers, in order for the big stores to book me. If you think about someone like Rosie Huntington-Whiteley who fronts the M&S lingerie campaign, that's what I'm talking about. This is the kind of gig Victoria wanted to secure for me. And I was happy to go along with it because I knew it meant big bucks and financial independence.

The question was: how do I get those bookings with magazines and newspapers as quickly as possible? New York was the most competitive city in the world for models and I needed to spread my wings. Where could I go where everyone speaks English? Victoria had a gleam in her eye as she said: 'London.' I was, as the Brits say, gobsmacked. Me? In London? Alone? Hell, yes. I could do this! And that's when the roller coaster ride *really* began…

* * * * * *

I arrived in London at the end of summer 1995. I watched the tiny, very green fields through the window as we came in to land and I thought it was absolutely beautiful, this kind of mythical country.

I can also clearly remember being wedged up against a very large British man on the eleven-hour flight. He was covered in tattoos and I thought, one day, I won't have to fly economy any more. I was sure I was headed for big things and that belief in myself stood me in good stead when I arrived in London. It needed to, believe me.

Victoria had arranged for me to be represented by a booking agent called Michelle at Select Models in London. Select were a huge agency; I was in great hands, but I was under no illusion that my look was fashion-forward at that time. Here I was, with my hips, my boobs, my butt and my bleached-blonde hair, competing with the urban-chic of Kate Moss and Chloë Sevigny with their anti-glamour style that was de rigeur, especially in London.

I needn't have worried because I found work immediately

and the bookings came thick and fast. Again, they weren't high fashion – the shoots offered to me were often lingerie and swimwear and then the German market started to take off and I began to get paid really good money to do catalogues for stores and brands over there. I spent just a few months in London, enough to find my feet, realise that this crazy, dirty city was exactly where I wanted to spend my life – at least for the foreseeable future – and I decided to fly home and say my goodbyes. Take me, London, I'm yours!

Chapter 3

The Day I Became Just 'Caprice'

I returned to London in early 1996 with the blessing of my mom, my sister and my agent, Victoria. I knew my destiny lay here; I wasn't sure how or what I was going to discover along the way but I knew I was going to make some money. And by now you'll know this was my driving force – it was never and never will be, about fame. It's all about money and my financial independence.

I moved into a room in Pimlico. A guy called Charles was renting his downstairs en suite bedroom. He was never there and the rent was cheap; it was an ideal situation. I didn't hang out with other models, generally, but I did meet some great people, including the stunningly gorgeous and very well-connected socialite, Tamara Beckwith. Tamara was lovely, and she took me under her wing. I don't really know why, because I found that, to begin with anyway, English people mocked us Yanks quite a lot. But Tamara and I had the same agent so I'm sure she had strict instructions from him to take me out and introduce me to her crowd.

During the mid 1990s, the whole concept of the 'Chelsea set' was really hot news and the public were fascinated, much as they are now, by the blue-blooded aristos and their lifestyles. I was seen as nouveau riche and some of the West London socialites looked down their noses at me, but I didn't let it bother me. Besides, it was around that time that a TV production company hit on the idea of what was to become one of the early reality TV shows: *Filthy Rich: Daddy's Girls*. And Tamara and I were both asked to be part of it. I'll comment more on the title of that show later, but I knew I'd be a fool not to give it a go.

Filming followed me, Tamara, and another girl called Charlotte as we lived our apparently glamorous lifestyles – off to the polo ('I was born to do this,' I say on camera at one point!), flying over to Paris, not to mention all the shopping we did. This was the prototype for today's *Made in Chelsea* with very much the same 'how the other half live' vibe.

I was fine with that, and we had a lot of fun making the show but for the fact I had no idea it was going to be called *Filthy Rich: Daddy's Girls* until later. When it aired, I was outraged. I was not a daddy's girl, or not in the way they meant it, and more than that, how dare they bring my dad into this. My mom had financed my upbringing and for my dad to somehow be credited as some kind of wealthy 'sugar daddy' who'd showered his daughter with cash all these years couldn't have been further from the truth.

There wasn't much I could do about the title, though, and the show did make quite a splash when it aired on Channel 4.

It was an interesting insight into an aspirational lifestyle and, alongside my modelling, it got me noticed – big time. Up until then I was pretty happy with the catalogue work I was doing, and I was making decent money. But before that show I was just another model and something of an 'it girl'.

In October that same year I was invited to present an award at the National TV Awards. It was the second year of the hot new awards show on ITV, which rewarded 'normal' TV for once – a soap might win an award as much as some grand BBC historical drama or super-serious documentary.

It was a huge event, held at the Royal Albert Hall. I hadn't been scheduled to go and I knew little about it but at the last minute my manager took a call from the producers. Clearly, one of their other guests had pulled out and they need a last minute replacement, but I didn't mind that one bit.

Wow. Just wow. This was a big one for me, in terms of great exposure to a really big TV audience. I didn't think twice before I said yes. Opportunities like this do not come along often – they didn't then and they're even harder to find now, since TV has been split into so many different channels.

I knew that the ratings for the show would be good because it was being televised on mainstream TV. All the great and the good from the TV world would be there, from national hero David Jason to the EastEnders and Coronation Street casts – even David Duchovny of the X-Files (I *loved* that show!) was nominated and rumoured to be over for the ceremony.

I had one day to find an outfit. The lovely Isabel Kristensen, a well-known society designer, offered to loan me a short, pink Barbie-doll style number. I loved it but I didn't think it was right. I'm not really a fluffy Barbie-doll type, I'm a little bit edgier than that. I went to a fashion PR agency and they offered to help me out but they only had three dresses they could loan me. As I looked over to the single rail in the corner of the room... well, I lost my breath. The first dress was perfect. It was long and made of black lace with a plunge neckline, with this sexy split up the side. It was Versace at his best. This was my 'it' dress.

I only had two hours to get home, get my hair and make-up done and dash out of the door to get to the awards ceremony. In the early years I didn't want to spend an astronomical amount to have a glam squad come in and make me look fabulous, so I did everything myself.

I took the dress carefully out of its tissue paper wrapping. I held it up to me and that's when it occurred to me: what the hell do I wear underneath this thing?

The top was fine as it was beautifully lined and had a sort of in-built bra – but the rest of the dress? Forget it. Nada, no lining. Completely and utterly see-through. I went through my underwear drawer and thank goodness I had one pair of lacy M&S undies. They had a few stray threads hanging from them but I had to make do. So I trimmed the threads and prayed they stayed intact for just one night. And so that's what I wore – a designer dress worth thousands of pounds teamed perfectly with a pair of well-worn knickers that I clearly should have thrown away two years before.

As I stepped out onto the red carpet, the photographers went completely wild. I'd never experienced anything like it, ever. And I absolutely loved it! It was so exciting, so thrilling to be the centre of all this attention. I knew then that this dress would do for me what Liz Hurley's 'safety pin' Versace gown had done for her, and that's exactly what happened.

Newsreader Trevor McDonald was hosting the awards that night and didn't quite know where to look when I came on stage to present the award. The papers went to town on him the next day for stumbling over his words and he later got into trouble with the TV bosses because he kept mentioning Wonderbra in relation to me and my – ahem – fairly well-displayed breasts!

Contrary to popular myth, I was never a Wonderbra model. That great honour from that time belongs firmly to Eva Herzigova for her stellar 'Hello Boys' campaign. The only thing I did was take part in the UK Wonderbra Week when I did a couple of photo shoots wearing their bras. I remember saying my boobs were insured for £50,000 at the time as a joke and, you know what? That line has followed me around ever since!

The awards night was thrilling and it went by in something of a blur. I didn't really know anyone so I just ran around the after-show party having a great time and talking to as many people as I could. All night, guys were following me around, hardly surprising when you're wearing a see-through dress, but I was the new girl on the block. The Yank with the boobs and the hair – and they loved it!

As fabulous as the NTV Awards were, I had no idea what effect the Versace dress would have. Next morning, sleepy-eyed and wearing whatever I'd just pulled on to nip to my local sandwich shop in Pimlico, I was woken out of my stupor by the man serving behind the counter asking for my autograph. Autograph? What, me?

Grinning from ear to ear, the guy showed me the front of *The Sun* newspaper, which had a big picture of me on it in the dress! I was plastered across all the national newspapers and I was dumbstruck when I saw it. I'd been going into that sandwich shop for four months and they'd never paid me special attention; now they were offering me free sandwiches!

I called my mom, I called my family and my friends, and everyone was screaming down the line at me. My boyfriend at the time, Robert T, a businessman I was totally in love with, was pretty thrilled too! It really was the best day of my life, I was so excited because this meant the big time and overnight I was transformed from being just a model into being a celebrity, and from then on, I was known in the press just by my first name.

The next 12 months were an absolute whirlwind for me. There was so much going on and I was working every single day. I spent long stretches of time on photo shoots for German catalogues, very often in places like Arizona, doing 12-hour days in the scorching heat, and they were really hard work, but I'd earn £24,000 for each job that took just ten days out of my life.

Sometimes we'd be in Mexico, other weeks it would be Germany, but we'd always stay in beautiful hotels and eat fantastic food. I think I was popular with the German market because it was hard to find blondes who looked strong and wholesome rather than trashy. It was lots of swimwear, lingerie and apparel.

Back in London between assignments, I'd earn £15,000 for doing a 45-minute personal appearance – this could be turning up to help promote anything from a new nightclub

50

to a boutique. And if they needed me for an extra 15 minutes then my manager would charge another £5,000.

I remember doing a promotional job for California Prunes during that year and I was paid something like £25,000 just to do a photo call – this is when all the newspaper journalists would turn up with their photographers, take a photo of me and I'd speak for a few minutes about California Prunes. It was utterly crazy, looking back.

I had my standards though – some jobs I wouldn't do, no matter how much was on offer. I'd just signed with a new talent agency called RDF Management who generally looked after my TV work, when my manager called me. 'Cap, we've had a very weird request but it means making £500,000 in half an hour.' Naturally, I was intrigued… but when it transpired that the request had come via a 'fixer' for a multibillionaire who wanted me to turn up to a party he was hosting – sit there, pretend I knew him, look impressed by the guy, then leave – I was not happy.

'So, if I turn up, everyone's going to know he's paid for me to be there – that is a totally different sort of profession! Forget it, I'm not interested,' I said.

My poor manager thought I was mad. 'Cap, we can make it clear to everyone what the situation is,' she said, exasperated by my stubbornness. But no matter how much I wanted to earn that kind of money, this would have ruined my reputation. The circles I was moving in were too small; it would risk everything just because a rich guy wanted his ego fed, wanting everyone to think I was there as his date.

I didn't need 'jobs' like that anyway. A year after the NTV Awards I'd made my first £1m and it was time to start putting that money to good use, and lay down the foundations for my future life.

The first thing I did when I started to make serious money was to buy my mom a house in Long Beach, not far from where I grew up in California. Mom had been living with relatives while she gradually got herself back on her feet and I knew having a permanent base was incredibly important to her.

I tried to be financially savvy about it though. I bought a place that was about to be repossessed and so it was a good price. I think I paid about $500,000 for it, which at that time was around £250,000. I spent some time in the summer helping Mom to do that place up. She really began to improve; I think having her own place and being creative again helped with her recovery. She was, after all, an interior designer and this was the perfect project for her.

I also bought a property in London, in a gated area of Fulham called Hurlingham Square, near the Thames. I doubled my money in just a couple of years. It was a great buy and it gave me the confidence to go into more property development.

During the late 1990s I started to buy properties, often in America. I'd generally hold onto them for two years (I was backwards and forwards between the US and UK all the time) and then I'd sell them on. This meant I avoided the US capital gains tax and taught me a lot about the market. Sometimes this would be a risk because I would pay out quite a bit of capital as a down-payment but nine times out of ten I would double on my investment and then put that money towards another property which cost more than the one I'd last paid for. I was upping the game each time.

Coming from a background where both of my parents had set up and run their own businesses, it was natural to me to be entrepreneurial and to look after my own finances.

There were projects I did that didn't necessarily bring in much money but were fun and interesting, and also about building my profile. I was being careful about my public image. I love a great time as much as anyone, but I had my feet on the ground. Though I partied a lot, I still wasn't a drinker; I was professional to my absolute core and I was really proud of that. The last thing I wanted was to be one of those celebs who are photographed falling out of a nightclub.

That appearance at the NTV Awards also led to an offer to play opposite Jonathan Ross in a TV commercial for Pizza Hut. At that time Pizza Hut had run a series of adverts with celebrities and sports personalities and in this 'episode' Jonathan and I had to pretend to be meeting at the restaurant on a first date, and I had to act as if I couldn't contain myself – I had to pretend to be completely in love with him and the fact that he couldn't say his 'Rs'.

I arrived on the day, nervous, a little excited and immediately blown away by the size of the set. It was huge! I hadn't expected this for a commercial but there were 40 people running around and it was all very Hollywood and glamorous. I thought, 'Holy smoke, this is all for me and Jonathan Ross? This is crazy.'

Jonathan just seemed quite used to it but I was staggered by it. It made me more nervous because I really wanted to do well. They were spending a lot of money on me so I didn't want to let anyone down. I was with Jonathan Ross and he was a big star!

It turned out that he was great to work with, and we had a ball making the commercial. Jonathan was very funny and generous to everyone on the shoot, from the cast to the crew, which was a nice surprise. Often you find with comedians that they're actually quite dour in real life, but Jonathan wasn't – he kept the banter up all the way through the filming and it was a real pleasure.

A few years later I also filmed a TV ad for Pot Noodle and that was great too. The campaign was all about misbehaving, and in one photo shoot I had to pretend to fall asleep whilst someone shaved all my hair off. Those pictures are hilarious!

Still riding off the back of the amazing Dress Success at the NTV Awards, 1998 was a fantastic year for me and my confidence was at an all-time high. I travelled so much and loved doing TV and I thought, I know, let's combine these two loves of mine and make my own TV show. I made a show reel with a production company and showed *Caprice's Travels* at the Cannes TV festival. The Travel Channel loved it and bought the show. Bingo! It was so great to be in right at the beginning of this process and for it to be my project; I loved it. It gave me a real taste for owning a product and was a great learning curve.

We had a tiny budget of £15,000 a show. It was tricky, but we made it work. We'd have around three days in each destination and I literally had to memorise the guide books to help me prepare for my pieces-to-camera. There wasn't a script, I just had to wing it! I would also interview people on the show and I really loved it, I met so many fascinating people on my travels.

In the end we made two series, each with ten episodes and it was pretty well received. We went all over the world from Blackpool (yes, I ate fish and chips!) to Mauritius. My absolute favourite was Jordan in the Middle East and the locations we saw for the movie *Lawrence of Arabia*. It was so stunning and the people were wonderful.

Working on *Caprice's Travels* gave me the opportunity to show people I wasn't just a model. I'm goofy, serious and self-deprecating in real life – and I guess I knew on some level it was a good idea for people to know the real me if I was going to stick around as a 'name' in the entertainment industry.

When you're at the top of your game, that's when you should be thinking about the next step. In many careers you can stay at the top of your industry for years, but as a model? No way. You have to think of Plan B *now*, not when things start falling off a cliff. I learned this early and it's a mantra I try to live by with everything I do.

I grew in confidence in terms of the risks I was willing to take with my photo shoots. There's a lot of very sexy, revealing pictures from that time, I can tell you! Because putting me on the cover was helping those publishers to sell their magazines, I started to call the shots a little bit. Not in an arrogant way but they let me have a lot of creative input.

I remember a GQ cover I did, when I asked for the photographer Willy Camden because I knew we worked really well together. I really wanted to push the limits. So I suggested to Willy, 'Let's do a shot where I'm looking over my shoulder, totally naked with my bare butt showing. I want you to bring out the whips and chains and let's go for it.' Of course Willy nearly wet himself and agreed without any hesitation.

It was a form of acting for me. I'd get into character and just run with it. The magazine editors knew they'd get their shot because I was doing this for my business as much as theirs.

On the sets it wasn't about flirting, it was about getting the best shots for the magazine and it felt so good to know I was in control. The atmosphere was just all about business. I look at some of those covers now and I'm so pleased I did them. Me in black masking tape? Check. Me ripping my lingerie off? Check. Me lying naked on a beach? Check! I knew the right shots were going to sell magazines and make the money to secure my future. I loved being in control of my life and I was doing what my mom had always taught me to do: making my own money.

The truth is, at that time of my life I loved taking my kit off because I felt sexy and I felt strong and I had control over what was happening. If people didn't like it then tough, I couldn't have cared less. As it was, people were actually pretty cool about it and my mom thought it was great! I'd send her the copies of the magazines and she'd show everyone: 'That's my daughter and she looks hot!'

In the late 1990s and the early 2000s the men's magazine market was thriving. *Loaded, FHM, Maxim* – all the men's monthly glossy titles were each selling at least half a million copies per issue and that was in the UK alone. And over the next few years, I appeared on around 200 covers, just in the men's market. I realised that if I retained the rights to the photographs, sharing the proceeds with the photographers, it would be pretty lucrative. A lot of the covers were used on the international issues of the magazines and I would usually have a contract drawn up to say the magazine could only use my image once and after that, the rights for the shoot would go back to the photographer. At that point, the photographer would go on to sell the pictures to every Tom, Dick and Harry, and make a fortune.

It dawned on me that I could make some money myself out of all those magazines I was helping to promote.

I couldn't believe there wasn't one celebrity at that time who didn't think about this. At that point in my career, I was allowed to choose the photographers I wanted, so I called up four of my favourites and said, 'Let's do a deal. I'll request you for the shoot but when you get the photographs back from the magazine, we'll do a split'.

At first most of them were reluctant but they came on board because if they didn't sign on the dotted line I'd have gone with another photographer who would. It was a brilliant idea because all I had to do was nine to ten cover shoots a year that would syndicate internationally and I made a fortune, well over six figures a year. I know this is common practice now but I can assure you no one was doing it back then.

I guess I was a bit of a pioneer at the time. I knew image worked for magazine readers so magazines needed me as much as I wanted their business.

They were crazy, fun times and every day was different. I'd fly to the most luxurious destinations for these cover shoots or to do a calendar, a lingerie or swimwear job. I was getting on a plane seven or eight times a month and I loved it. One day I'd be in the Seychelles in the warm, turquoise waters of the Indian Ocean, the next I'd be on a private yacht in Nice. I had a glamorous life for sure, but I knew it wouldn't last forever and that's why I worked so hard and tried as much as possible to think out of the box in terms of making deals.

When I look back at pictures from that time, I see these stunning, sexy, windblown shots of me in exotic places like the Mojave Desert in California and I can't help recalling the circumstances of the shoots. I mean, there it was either boiling hot and over 100°F – even in January it can get that high, or freezing cold because once the sun goes down the wind howls around you and you freeze your ass off.

They were long days, starting around sunrise and we'd carry on shooting most of the day because it would save on costs. The less time we stayed away from the UK, the less the magazine or catalogue would have to spend. They were great days though, with hard-working teams who would all pull together to make the pictures work.

I was riding high, but I was making sure I was careful with my money. I was a saver, always have been. I mean, I bought myself my first Mercedes. They're my favourite cars even now. I'd rent a yacht with friends if we were partying for a weekend so yes, there would be blow-outs, but in all other ways I watched the pennies. I never flew first class if I was paying because it was stupidly expensive! I trained my PA at the time to get all the best deals on business class or use my air miles to buy an economy ticket and bump me up: 'Go to this travel agent first,… what's my best option?' But the days of flying economy class were behind me!

While all this was happening, I still had my West London party-girl friends and Tamara and I were still close, but I lived alone and there were no serious boyfriends in my life. Robert T and I had gone our separate ways by this point. The truth was, I didn't have time to invest in relationships of any kind because I just wasn't around enough. When I think about the wide circle of friends I now have, it's quite strange to look back on how isolated I was in some ways, but I didn't feel I needed people: I was very, very focused on making my career work for me, on my terms. That's still important, but with that kind of drive often comes loneliness. No one gets close to you, because by necessity you're self-absorbed. These days I'm much more about the people I love. And I like to think I'm a nicer person for it.

I will say this for back then, though: I did feel a little bit judged by people in my set – the Chelsea It crowd. I knew they disapproved of me, maybe because I was a Yank, but I was never a bitch or a gossip, and if I could I would always take care of anyone who needed it. I may not have been what the It crowd thought of as a girly girl, but I was always decent to those around me.

Mom has always had a lot of integrity. She's good to people and I was raised to be the same. I was rebellious and a bit wild but I treated everyone with respect whether they were a janitor or a billionaire. Striking that balance back then was a challenge and it took my plummet from grace to teach me that I needed girlfriends around me for support.

What I've learned is that it's really hard, when so many people around you are telling you how amazing you are, not to start believing a little too much in your own hype – especially when you're in your twenties and believe you're invincible. I'll be the first one to admit that my ego was getting a little bit out of control. Everywhere I went people were like:

'Yes, Caprice, of course you can have that, you're wonderful, we love you, you're gorgeous ...' and I believed them.

My house was always full of flowers and chocolate, thank-you gifts for photo shoots or jobs I'd done, or from admirers trying their luck. I got used to it. I had no responsibilities and so I just went with the flow and had fun.

I cringe when I think of the diva I was at times, though. My wonderful PA Vicky was with me throughout this period and I'd often say to her, 'Let's go to this hot new club.' I'd make her call up the club and say: 'Caprice wants to come to the club tonight, we want ten bottles of vodka and we're bringing ten people and we want it for free.'

Sometimes they'd say no – and she'd do the whole, 'Do you know who we're talking about?' I mean! How embarrassing is that? If Vicky wasn't successful with one club, she'd call up another until she got what she wanted. At the time I loved Vicky's arrogant behaviour, but now I think we both look back and cringe.

I'd also taken to asking for the clothes I wore on shoots. What's more, I'd want them for free! Poor Vic would have to call them up and ask them. There was no one to bring me back down to earth again – except my mom. If she was with me and she overheard my phone calls she'd say, 'You're just a middle-class girl from Hacienda Heights, give me a break. Who the hell do you think you are?' But I only half-listened to her then; I thought I was so cool and I knew it all.

I wasn't mean or unkind, I was just somewhat full of myself. When I think back to that time now, and the subsequent events in my life, I believe that karma and the universe never lets you get away with things completely. Later on, when I got into a bit of trouble, I couldn't help but wonder if life was teaching me a valuable lesson.

During this period I was often asked onto TV shows. I was a guest presenter on *The Big Breakfast* alongside Jonny Vaughan for a week, I acted on a show called *Dream Team* (I was so bad, what was I thinking?) and I remember just before Christmas 1999, filming an episode of *Bang, Bang, It's Reeves and Mortimer*, which went out on New Year's Day. I've watched this back since and I can tell you, I couldn't understand a damn word they were saying! Vic and Bob have such strong Geordie accents and I was this all-American girl just nodding along with everything they said and looking really vacuous because I just couldn't understand them!

Chapter 4

Hello Boys

I may not have wanted a serious relationship with anyone, but that didn't stop me dating left, right and centre. I just wanted to go out and have fun. If it stopped being fun, then we'd just agree to part and I'd move on and there were no dramas. I was just happy jumping around from one relationship to the next. And, apart from that I didn't have time for anything heavy, my first experience of dating a British guy had made me a little wary of the men I was meeting here...

Back when I was on one of my very first trips to London I met a man – let's call him 'Steven' (you'll understand why it's not his real name shortly) – and we dated for a couple of months. I had to fly out for a photo shoot for one of my German catalogues so I was away for a couple of days.

Steven called me to say, 'Hey, Cap, why don't I meet you at your hotel when you get back from your job?' Steven already had my room key from a previous visit and so when the plane landed, I headed straight to see him. I went up in the lift, looking forward to a night of passion with my man. The sight that met my eyes was enough to stop anyone in their tracks. There was Steven, top-to-toe in lingerie – *my* lingerie – and, to add insult to injury, he was wearing my best Louis Vuitton shoes, which he'd stretched horribly across his big, manly feet and he was rubbing his nipples through the lacy bra that was stretched across his hairy chest.

I watched him quietly – he didn't know I was there at first because it was dark in the room. And then suddenly, before my eyes, this guy started to pull something out of his ass. And whatever it was, they were glow-in-the-dark and they were green. Stephen had actually inserted some really big anal balls into his ass and was pulling them out as he played with himself – and all of this whilst wearing my lingerie!

He suddenly realised that I was in the room but instead of looking embarrassed, he looked calmly over at me and said, 'Don't you think I look good?' And all the while he was playing with his nipples! I wasn't even *slightly* tempted to play along, I was kind of horrified. Funnily enough, I'd never seen anyone pull glow-in-the-dark balls out of their ass before. Stephen didn't seem remotely worried at what I might think; he was quite blasé about the whole thing and even suggested I join him.

It was very, very late at night and I was dog-tired. At that point in my life I'd only been romantic with a few boys and so I thought, maybe this is normal behaviour here in England. So rather than kicking him out, I spent a very tense night waiting for him to leave. I didn't return his calls after that.

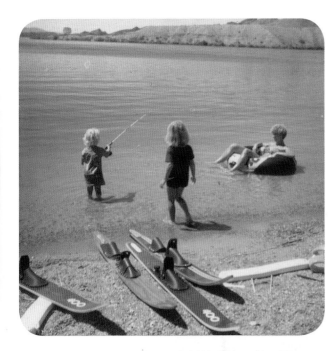

Left: My sister, my mum and I at Lake Havasu in 1975.

Below: My sister, our ski instructor and I in Mammoth California, in 1980.

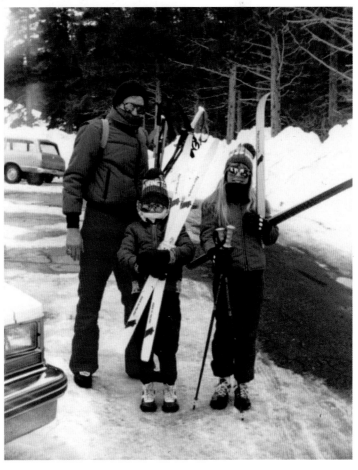

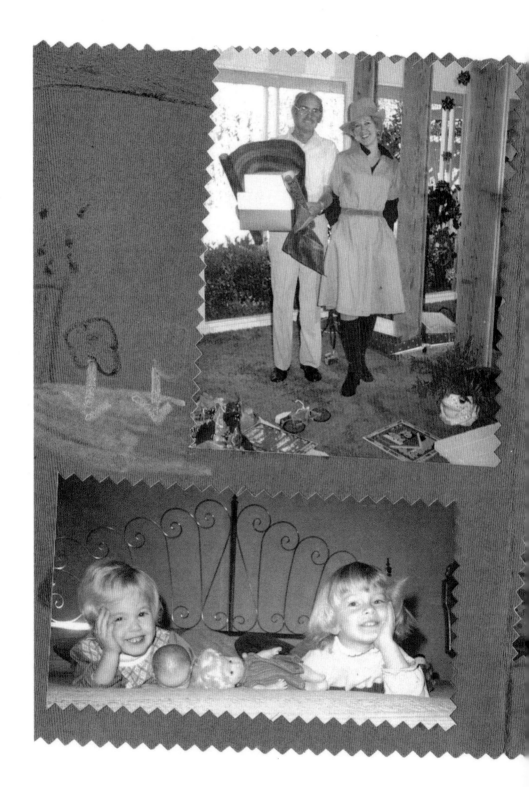

Above: Papa, Tippy, Mom and I in 1974.

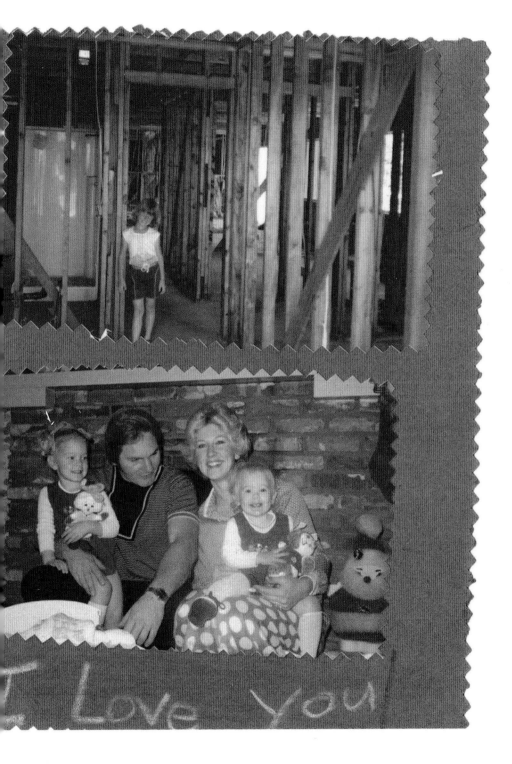

I Love You

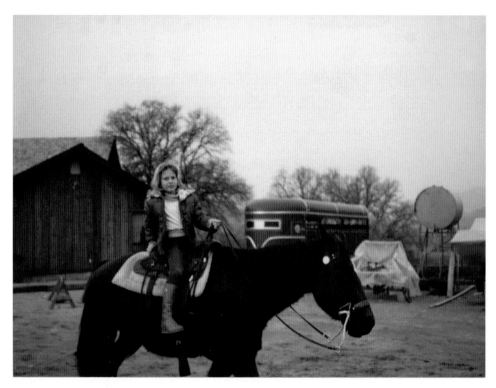

Above: Hawaii, in 1980... yep that's me.

Below: My sister and cousin in 1984.

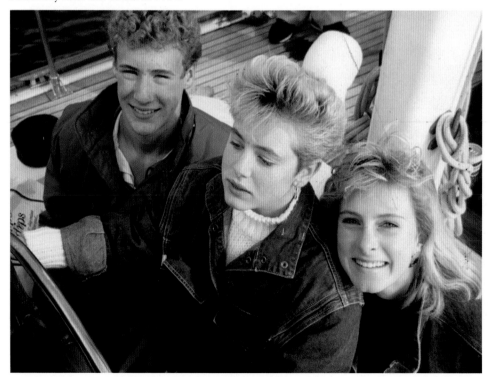

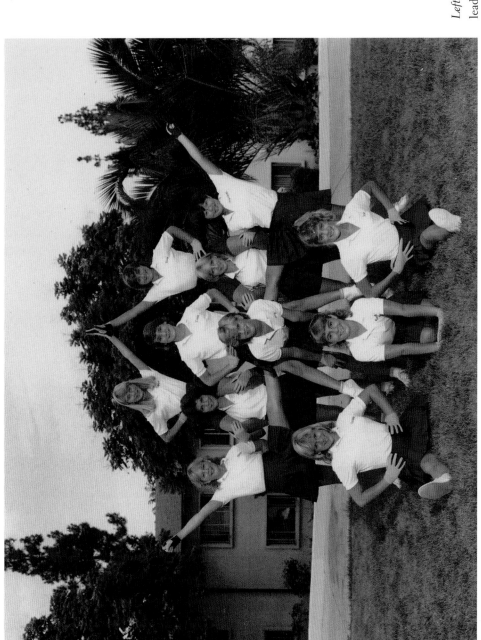

Left: My Junior High cheer-leading squad and I in 1985.

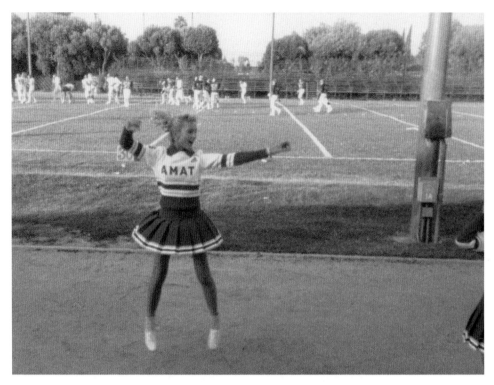

Above: A shot of myself in my sophomore year in 1987.

Below: My mom took a picture of me with my brand new
Dynastar skis in our living room on my 16th birthday in 1988.

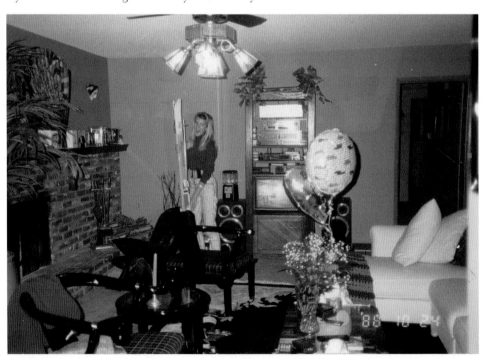

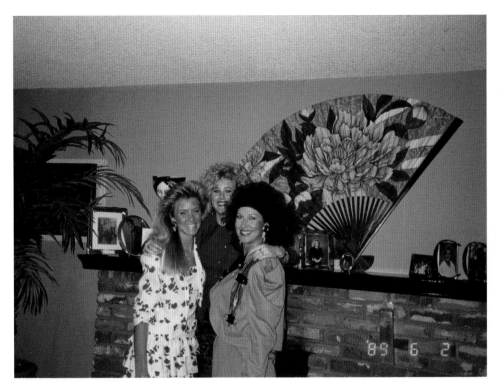

Above: Tippy, mom and I in 1989.

Below: Annette and I collecting our cheerleading
trophy from the Dallas Cowboy cheerleaders in 1989.

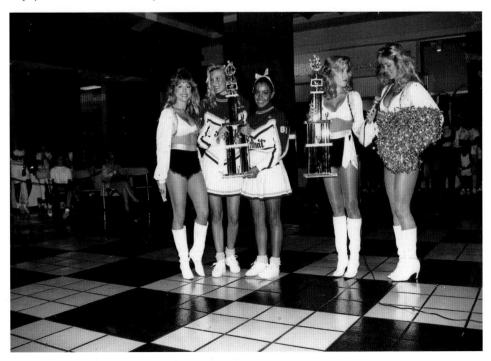

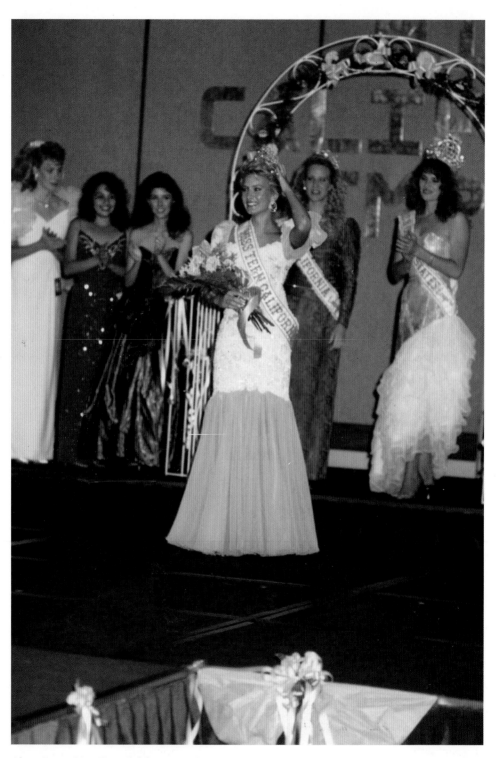

Above: I won Miss Teen California in 1989.

The whole thing was so bizarre that I couldn't wait to get on the phone to my mom and tell her what had happened.

'Mom! You'll never believe it, I don't think I can stay in this country. English men are just so weird.' I told her the story and she was absolutely horrified. She told me to get on a plane immediately and come home. That was a little bit dramatic; of course I didn't get on a plane and go home. In fact, a few years on from this, all had changed. I wasn't a little sweet innocent girl from Hacienda Heights any more – oh, what a little bit of fame and financial independence can do to a girl. By that time my confidence levels had gone through the roof, I was taking full advantage of my new life, I was in my mid twenties, not bad looking, rich and famous. A recipe for complete disaster.

I remember flying into Las Vegas to do a PA (personal appearance) and I'd called up my friends from LA to come with me. We were up in the VIP balcony overlooking the nightclub and there were probably around 1,500 people, a crowd mostly made up of very good-looking men. I'd say, 'OK, girls, which ones do you want this evening?' And they'd look incredulously at me and say, 'Cap, what are you on?'

'Go on,' I'd insist. 'Pick a guy you want to hang out with tonight; the bouncer will go get him and bring him up here.' And that would be it. Usually the guys would be thrilled to accommodate. Can you imagine how arrogant I was in those days? It's just ridiculous!

Nobody could believe it – women behaving like men? That never happened. But it was all just fun, the boys had a great time and so did we.

Sure, I liked a man to hunt me; it made me feel empowered. Not to sound arrogant, but I had flowers delivered to
me every single day from one guy or another, to the point
that it started to mean nothing. So, if a guy did something
different I'd sit up and take notice.

I remember meeting someone at a party who asked me
what my favourite chocolate bar was. I said Snickers and a
few days later I opened my front door to find 150 Snickers
bars arranged in a heart on my front door step! It made me
smile, even though it wasn't enough to make me go out with
him. My head was getting bigger and bigger by the day.

I may have been playing the field, but I definitely wasn't a
cold bitch who had no feelings. I just enjoyed being in that
permanent honeymoon stage – when you're both on your
best behaviour and trying everything to impress. As soon as
that changed, I got out. I guess deep down, when it came to
sex and real intimacy I was always quite shy and cautious. So,
no – I wasn't sleeping my way around London. One night
stands were never my 'thing'. If they were, I would happily
tell you, but I loved the chase and the longer they chased
me, the better.

Throughout this period, I didn't really drink any alcohol;
that didn't happen until my late twenties. As soon as you hit
the public eye, your behaviour is scrutinised. I'd had my fair
share of press exposure – and the last thing I wanted was to
add to the gossip. Call it control, call it self-preservation, but
not drinking kept my head clear and my reputation intact. I
believe in taking responsibility for your behaviour, and press
coverage works both ways.

My confidence was definitely shattered towards the end of

1998, though. I was riding high on the success of my career and I was having an absolute blast. I'd been working on a photo shoot all day and decided to go straight over to the house of the guy I was seeing at the time. I was just about to get in the bathtub in his bathroom when I saw a long brown hair in the tub.

I climbed out, walked slowly up to him and casually dangled the hair in front of his face. 'Would you like to explain who this belongs to?' I asked. He flushed guiltily and made up some ridiculous lie about it being his cleaner's hair. Now let me make it very clear to you: his cleaner had short, black, frizzy hair on her head. There is no way this two-feet-long piece of brown hair could have belonged to her. I had already heard from my friends that he was cheating on me and hadn't wanted to believe it. But now I did. He twisted the situation around and told me I was just neurotic. That manipulative, mind-game stuff might work on other women but not me. I was out of there. I broke up with him and never looked back, never even contemplated it. I think I would have had more respect for him if he'd just told me the truth. After all, I wouldn't have blamed him. I was never around because I was always away on catalogue trips.

At this point, no one I'd dated had been in the public eye. I usually went out with guys I'd met through friends. Then I started working with Ian Wright on his hot new chat show, *Friday Night's All Wright*. Ian was something of a legend – he was an England player and had been with Arsenal for seven years when he landed the show and it was a massive success. It had the all-important 10.30pm slot on a Friday night and regularly garnered 4m viewers. Ian was known for being really good fun and a little bit cheeky.

The first time I appeared it was to talk about *Caprice's Travels* but, honestly? We didn't talk much about that. 'Wrighty', as he's known, just wanted to find out what it was like posing in swimwear and living a glamorous supermodel life, and he loved taking the mickey out of me – and I gave as good as I got! Ian and I got on so well I appeared in the rest of the series as his 'doorman' and it was my job to introduce the guests. I played up the dumb blonde – but with a nod to the audience. I knew what was going on!

Ian liked to invite his mates onto his show as much as anyone who had a single or movie to promote. The format wasn't as serious as *Parkinson* had become, and it was an era that was ripe with new talent. One week it would be the Appleton sisters from All Saints, the next it might be Janet Jackson, but it would always be someone who was prepared to have some fun on the show. A sort of precursor to Graham Norton's style, I guess.

One of Ian's guests was footballer Tony Adams. And can I say what a beautiful, 6ft 4 hunk of a guy he was! I introduced him with the words: 'He's tall, he's dark and he's absolutely gorgeous.' Tony was the England football team captain and captain of Arsenal and was on a roll. That year Arsenal had won the Premiership and the FA Cup – which I have to ad-mit, didn't mean an awful lot to me – I just recognised that this man was special.

Tony had gone through some pretty tough times and a well-documented struggle with alcoholism but those days were behind him and I found him to be a true gentleman.

Ian ribbed him about the fact that he was learning to play the piano and becoming something of a bookworm, which at that time surprised me. I wasn't very up on footballers but I suppose I assumed they weren't necessarily the sharpest knives in the cutlery drawer. But how wrong I was about Tony.

He wasn't traditionally good-looking but he was very, very sexy. He seemed understated, everything about him from his style through to his way of expressing himself. So we flirted a little on the show and I thought, wow, he's hot, but we went our separate ways.

A few days later, I was about to go into a restaurant called Halepi when my phone rang.

'Who is this?' I asked cautiously. It was an unknown number and I don't usually answer those calls. 'It's Tony Adams, I met you on Ian's talk show. Would you like to go out some time?'

I was so taken aback I just said, 'I know who you are and I can't believe you're calling me!' Of course, I said yes because I already had a crush on him. We started dating each other in late 1998 and the relationship was kept very private at first.

Tony and I were sneaking around, trying not to get spotted together and, I have to admit, it was very exciting! We didn't exactly go out in disguise but we went to some very quiet restaurants and sneaked into out-of-the-way movie theatres to avoid detection. We both had such huge profiles at this stage and so to see the two of us together would be tabloid heaven.

In the end, we were busted smooching near a movie theatre in the back streets of Piccadilly. I remember the picture well – we were leaning against a big pole and I was reaching up to kiss him wearing my white sneakers, brown leather jacket and jeans. That was the shot and it went everywhere. The story was out and the circus began.

Within days *Hello!* magazine had called us and offered a crazy amount – like, seven digits – for the wedding. I thought, hold on a minute, we've only been dating each other for two seconds! We were the hottest couple of the moment and I'll admit I loved it!

Tony was used to press following him everywhere. Some of the time they were waiting for him to misbehave because at that stage he hadn't been sober for long. And so our relationship certainly piled on the pressure in terms of the publicity he was getting. Wherever we went, we were photographed and followed. We would see people listening into our conversations in restaurants and although I was enjoying the attention, I could tell that he wasn't so into it. I felt it wasn't healthy for him to have this extra attention at this stage in his life.

Tony was a very focused, honourable person. He was still working through his demons after struggling with alcoholism, and Arsene Wenger, the Arsenal manager, was a big support to him. Whenever Tony had a game, he wouldn't see me beforehand because he needed to really focus on the match. I really hated it when he wouldn't see me. Or maybe it was my ego talking and as a result I felt rejected. I look back on it now and I think, how cringeworthy was that?

I had genuinely fallen for Tony but I'm not going to pretend that I didn't enjoy the fact that we were the biggest celebrity couple of the moment. The model and the footballer – this was way before WAGS were invented as a 'thing', and Victoria and David Beckham had only just started dating. The paparazzi photographers (paps) would be following us around constantly – jumping out of bushes, turning up outside restaurants. But Tony was much more humble about his status in the public eye than I was.

One morning during this time, Tony called me and asked if I was at home. He said he needed to come to see me immediately. And as soon as I opened the door and looked at him, I knew what he was going to say. 'Cap, I just can't do this any more.' Without going into detail, we both knew that the time wasn't right for us. Both of us had so much going on, we weren't seeing a lot of each other and being thrown to the paps at this point wasn't too healthy for Tony.

I understood, but I was pretty upset. I shut the door behind him and I buried my heartache in songwriting. I felt rejected and it was the first hard knock I'd had in my love life.

A few months prior to this, in 1999, I'd been offered a record deal with Virgin, which was a huge thrill to me. I was beyond delighted. Remember the strategy? Build on what you have while the going's good? This was part of the strategy and anyway, I thought it would be fun to try something completely different. I wanted to act and sing – in fact, building a career on stage was something I was really keen to pursue. I wanted to create music I liked dancing to and I was writing my own material. Something with a great beat, catchy hooks and lyrics which actually meant something to me – nothing frivolous, they had to have meaning.

I was upset about my break-up with Tony but my A&R guy at Virgin told me to write about it. 'Cap, when you're down, this is when you write the good stuff,' he said. And so I wrote a song called 'The Idea of Being in Love'. It's all a bit cheesy but most of the pop songs during that era were really cheesy.

After the break-up, it was months before Tony and I had any contact and it gave me some time to think about the kind of girlfriend I'd been. Tony's life had been in turmoil for some years and just as he was really straightening things out, I'd brought my demands out: I wanted him to be at my beck and call. I wanted him to go to dinner parties when I organised them; I wanted him to go to events with me and when he couldn't or wouldn't, I took it really personally. I loved the fact that people were interested in us as a couple but he didn't. I understood what had happened and why, but I was still sad. And I really didn't want the whole of England reading about the break-up but it wasn't long before the story leaked out to the media.

Luckily, the press were pretty decent about it and said the decision had been 'mutual', with both of us too busy to commit properly to a relationship. It was time for me to lick my wounds and get on with my life.

My first single, 'Oh Yeah', was due out shortly after the split and I concentrated on promoting that, which meant travelling around the country a lot and sometimes performing to audiences of around 30,000 people. I did a whole series of road shows where I'd go to a different venue every single night for about a month. I loved it! I went up and down the UK – over to Ireland, up to Scotland, although I remember the best response seemed to be from the audiences in Manchester and Birmingham, where they'd go crazy.

Sometimes I'd do two gigs a night – each with 2,000 people in the audience and I did festivals all over the country too. I was on a high – this was me reinventing myself, trying something different – and I loved it. The single sold

30,000 copies, which back then got me to number 24 in the charts – now that would probably be enough to hit number one.

One of the nights I did, which was great fun, was at G.A.Y. – the legendary gay club in central London, which always attracted a huge and enthusiastic crowd.

I had a surprise guest that night – Rod Stewart had asked to be put on my guest list along with a mutual friend of ours. Rod was 54, I was 27 and it was about a year after he'd split up with his wife, Rachel Hunter. Everyone knew how heart-broken he'd been and I think he was just getting back into dating. We met for the first time when my friend brought Rod backstage at the end of the night. I was surprised – I hadn't realised he was very witty and self-deprecating, and that drew me to him. I wasn't sure if I fancied him but I knew I really liked him.

Straight after the gig I was flying out to Puerto Rico to film a TV series called *Dream Team*. It was a sort of US remake of *Charlie's Angels* and it aired in 1999.

Whilst I was out there filming, Rod called me to see if I'd like to go out on a date when I was back in the UK. Well, I wasn't going to turn down dinner with a superstar like Rod Stewart. I remember him coming to pick me up from my house in Hurlingham Square and he arrived in something terribly glamorous like a Ferrari (funny, I'd always made fun of men in fast cars ... you know what they say!) but I couldn't help but be impressed.

The papers went into overdrive again, just as they had with Tony. But this was different. I think Rod quite liked the press attention and we all now know I loved it as well ...

Later on I flew out to LA and Rod, who was already over there, picked me up from the airport and drove me to Long Beach to meet my mom. I think she was star-struck. I got the impression she might have had a crush on him, many years ago.

He took me to his house, where I met his kids. I don't think the children liked me very much because the first time I walked into the house I noticed that there wasn't a picture in sight of Rod with another woman – not one amongst the thousands of pictures all over the house. But the following day, out of nowhere, the whole house was suddenly decorated with pictures of him and Rachel Hunter. Even on top of the toilet there was a picture of Rachel! I can't blame the children; I probably would have done the exact same thing. After that, Rod flew back to England and I stayed in LA for another month. I remember calling him and oddly not getting a return call, which was definitely not like him. And from that day on, I never heard from him again.

Well, at least if I had to get dumped by a man twice my age, it was by Rod Stewart.

Chapter 5

The Fun Continues

In London, I was still hanging out with the Chelsea set, who made it their business to have as much fun as possible – especially at weekends. Most of them had homes in the country, and a group of us would often go out for the weekend and engage in country pursuits: clay pigeon shooting, picnics, long very boozy lunches… it was a great way to make more friends!

I remember one house in particular, Sherborne Castle in Dorset. It was stunningly beautiful and you could feel the history permeating through the walls. It had been the home of Sir Walter Raleigh in the 17th century and a house had been standing there since the 12th century. There was a party of around 20 of us all there one weekend and I remember one of the girls saying, 'Come on, let's have a séance.' I wasn't going to let a little thing like ghosts spook me.

It was the first time I'd taken part in a séance – I'd always thought it was something slightly bonkers that people did in Victorian times. I had no idea people took it seriously, but I was up for the experience. Why not?

We all gathered around a table in a circle whilst our host (who'd clearly done this a few times before) called up the spirits of the dead – in this case, Sir Walter Raleigh. He kept saying the name over and over again and then, suddenly, all the lights went out and the whole room froze. I mean that literally – we were all absolutely freezing, the air was cold and the hairs on the back of my neck stood up in a way I'd never experienced. It lasted for around two minutes, which is a very long time if you're in the dark. Then the lights went back on and normal service was resumed. But it was enough to freak me out. I loved the crowd I was with, and there were a couple of interesting men I was just getting to know that weekend, but even they were not gorgeous enough to keep me in that house a minute longer. I retired as quickly as possible to a nearby hotel and never went back.

I found out afterwards that Sherborne is known for its hauntings, possibly by the ghost of Sir Walter Raleigh. I'm no believer in the paranormal, but something happened that night, I'm sure of it, and that place is officially creepy.

It also put paid to any romantic developments that particular weekend, but I was moving in circles that brought me into contact with such a wide variety of people. I loved British men because I found them to be honest and courteous. None more so than royalty!

I met Prince Andrew through some mutual friends, and we exchanged numbers but there was never a romance there.

Prince Andrew is a charming, witty, well-travelled man and the fact that he's a prince is not important – well, until the rumour is out that you're supposedly dating him! I haven't talked about this period of my life very much until now because really, there isn't much to say. He and I were just good mates and that's as far as I wanted it to go. I think if I was going to date someone in the public eye I wanted to date a rock star not a prince – that's a little too 1950s for me.

He's very grounded and normal considering the extraordinary life he's led. Whenever we met, it was usually for dinner at restaurants like The Lanesborough where we knew they were discreet and we wouldn't be surrounded by photographers.

Nothing stays discreet for long, though. One evening I was invited, along with some of Andrew's other friends, to the palace where he had a flat at the time. We had a fabulous dinner, waited on by footmen and drinking vintage champagne, but the next day the story was out. He thought it was probably one of the guards at the palace who'd leaked it but that was it. Bang. We were 'the prince and the showgirl' to the newspapers.

My mom was straight on the phone. 'You're making the news over here in the States, Cap! What do you mean you're not actually going out with him? Why not?'

But much as I liked Prince Andrew, I didn't have those kind of feelings for him. I thought he was a lovely man and still do. The papers misinterpreted the relationship entirely, and as soon as that happened it became uncomfortable for me so we stopped communication.

I was still only 29 years old and making more and more TV appearances – including stints on *The Big Breakfast*, standing in for Denise Van Outen while she was away. I also secured an incredible gig hosting *An Evening at the Oscars* for the ABC Network in America as well as the American Music Awards (AMAs) where I presented the live red carpet feed for both shows. ABC loved me at the time.

Events like the AMAs and the Oscars have a colossal global audience and being asked to work on these shows was a dream come true and sometimes I really didn't believe it was happening to me. I think maybe I coped with it by just keeping busy and not actually thinking about it too much, although my ego hadn't got any smaller, that's for sure.

When I look back I guess it was the pinnacle of everything I'd been working towards as a model. My modelling career had taken me into exciting new projects and I was learning how to present and perform in front of a live camera and it gave me a taste for acting, which I'd develop more in a few years' time. I'd even starred in a documentary – all about me! It was called *Being Caprice* and was made by Emily Fielden, a friend I'd worked with before on other projects. The show aired on Channel 4 in the summer of 2000 and it was another early reality TV show, just as reality TV as we now know it started to really take off.

I agreed to wear a camera for ten days and the idea was that you'd get a glimpse into the life of a supermodel. It was challenging to do because I was meant to keep the camera on virtually 24/7 and in the end, the 30-minute documentary was a snapshot of my life –from riffling through my knicker drawer to stepping out of the car and onto the red carpet at the Brits. The British press can be pretty harsh but I think at that time they realised there was a growing hunger for this kind of show and they were surprisingly kind.

The Guardian said: 'Being Caprice could have been cheap and trashy, but its insights are surprisingly subtle and dark. The abiding impression one has of Caprice is of a woman surrounded by silent, staring men: from door security and bodyguards to TV producers, photographers, and, of course, her fans.'

I'm not sure I agree with their take on my life but all the same, it felt like this show, at that time, was going to be too intimate, too revealing for me to be comfortable with continuing and so it stayed a one-off documentary. Still, it meant those early tastes of reality TV had whetted my appetite. I wasn't afraid of appearing in shows like Celebrity Big Brother later down the line, mainly because I wasn't scared of people seeing me for who I am.

There was a downside to all of this though, in that the press didn't just hound me (which I could handle and quite enjoyed) but they wouldn't leave my mom or my sister alone either. They were forever harassing them for stories. My mom would be at a traffic stop light and a journalist would get out and start taking pictures of her; if she went out with no make-up on the papers would say horrible things about her. At other times they'd call her or other members of the family and pretend to be a friend of mine, trying to get information out of them about whom I was dating. She really wouldn't ever want to go through that again.

For now, events, parties and presenting were all part of my whirlwind life, alongside the photo shoots and the advertising campaigns. I remember heading to the MTV Europe

Awards in Rotterdam where I was to present an award. It was a very eventful night!

It was 8th November 2001 and I'd had a very early start for a photo shoot for the cover of *You* magazine, the *Mail on Sunday*'s influential weekly women's title. Afterwards I flew straight from London to Frankfurt. I had three cars pick me up from the door of the aeroplane. My bags were put into the boot and I was off. I only had 20 minutes to get to Rotterdam as I was due to go on stage in an hour.

I had a police escort in front of me, I had a police escort behind; I felt like I was the goddamned president of the United States. We hit speeds of 150 miles an hour to get me there in time. When I arrived, I was whisked off to my dressing room with only 45 minutes to get ready before I hit the stage with my gorgeous co-presenter, Aerosmith legend Steven Tyler. As I walked into my dressing room a cloud of smoke billowed forth and as it cleared, there, in all her cream and gold finery, sat Missy Elliott.

'Come on in, baby doll' husked Missy, patting the seat next to her. Missy was enjoying the fame and adulation which came with having a huge hit. 'Get Ur Freak On' was that year's anthem and she was queen bee. Sharing a dressing room with Missy came halfway through one of my kid-in-a-candy-shop days – a day which had begun with a glamorous photo shoot and ended with me setting the gossip columns on fire (again).

Missy peered at me through the smoke. Man, she had a presence! I was struck dumb. I pretended to be cool but the day was getting surreal. I'd left home ten hours earlier, worked my ass off on a shoot, jumped on a plane, flown halfway across Europe and now my new bestie was Missie freakin' Elliott. Holy smoke, things couldn't have got any better.

After five minutes in make-up I was bundled onto the stage and thrust into the spotlight next to the enigmatic (and sexually frenetic) Mr Tyler. Those lips were *big*! 'Cappy, you look hot in that dress,' he whispered, just before we stepped on stage. Know what? I've kept that dress. How could I not after a compliment from him? Steven Tyler might have been getting on in years but he was still hot! (Don't worry, I wasn't about to do another Rod Stewart – those days were gone.)

The night belonged, however, to Limp Bizkit. The nu metal band won three awards and lead singer Fred Durst was on a high. Fred and I hung out that entire night. At one point, someone came over to ask me for my autograph and didn't even look at Fred, who then looked at me, pretty bemused, and said: 'How did that happen?' At the time Fred and his band were riding high, whereas I was 'just' a model. I'm not going to lie. It was a great moment!

Our unlikely match gave the gossip columnists a whole lot to talk about for the next few days. Fred is a really sweet guy and he'd recently split with his long-term girlfriend. We had a lot in common, plus he's really sexy – especially if you like tattoos. Thankfully this was before the days of social media because a match like that would have sent Twitter into meltdown had it happened in 2015.

At the time, I was dating an actor and comedian called David Spade. David had made his name on *Saturday Night Live* in the US and was pretty big news over there. Then he was starring in a show called *Just Shoot Me*, but I met him at a club in LA when a friend of his came over to say, 'David Spade would like to meet you.'

Unfortunately, I had no idea who he was! I'm afraid the first words out of my mouth were, 'Is he hot?' His friend laughed hysterically and said, 'Yeah, he's really hot.' I couldn't understand why his friend was laughing so much; it wasn't a funny question. I quickly found out why when I met Dave – he came up to my nose and definitely wasn't a looker. But he was so damned funny. At first we just hung out together a lot and even after a few months I wasn't sure if we should officially be in a relationship. He was very smart and eccentric and he made me laugh all the time.

Fred Durst called me the day after the MTV Europe Awards and said, 'I'm in New York and I'd like to see you. I'm sending you a ticket – if you get on the plane, great. If you don't, whatever.' Oh my god, now *this* doesn't happen very often. A hot rock star sending me a first class return trip ticket to New York, just so he could take me to lunch. But I was sort of seeing Spade. What was a girl to do? Well, get on the plane, of course.

I felt a little bit guilty. It was really naughty, but I was so carried away with the moment I didn't consider the consequences. I'm not someone who cheats and I was just being a little bit silly, but I guess my justification was that David and I weren't in a serious relationship so it was fine. And it was just lunch, anyway.

I flew to New York the next day, jittery and excited about what I was doing; it felt so crazy. I was picked up by Fred's driver and taken to the Four Seasons hotel, where Fred was also staying (but I had my own room, I hasten to add) to check in before I went to meet him at La Goulou, a fabulous French restaurant on Madison Avenue.

We pulled up outside the restaurant and, lo and behold, there were about 50 paparazzi photographers. I don't know how they knew we were coming, but they knew. Maybe Fred had made the reservation under his own name and someone from the restaurant had tipped them off, but what it meant was that we were in for a very unrelaxing meal.

The paps sat outside our window trying to get a picture until, in the end I had to ask them to shut the curtains during lunch. It was so obnoxious. I mean, I loved the attention but this was a step too far. Conversation flowed and we had a great time but I did have to mention the fact that I was seeing someone and it might be better if we left the restaurant separately. A little bit of shutting the door after the horse has bolted, I realise, but still, I tried.

I think he was a bit insulted after I told him we had to leave separately. He later told me he had to go to a recording session and his driver would take me back to the hotel. We'd have dinner later that night.

I was not happy. I was fuming in fact. I'd flown across the world (OK, at his expense, but still) to see him and now I had to sit in a hotel room waiting for Mr Bizkit to make it back from his recording session. I honestly thought, 'Fuck this, I'm off home.' I called his assistant and said, 'I'll pay for my own ticket home and make sure Fred's reimbursed from the airline. Thanks very much for lunch, goodbye.' I flew out that evening.

And that was it, we never spoke again. To be honest, I think we were going neck and neck in the ego race! He was probably thinking, 'What the fuck, no one does that to me!' and I was thinking, 'What the fuck, no one does that to *me!*' I thought he was an attractive guy but there's no way I was going to hang around for anyone like that. I had far too much pride and, anyway, it was a very rude thing to do!

David Spade never did find out about my flying visit to New York to see Fred. It's been a secret – until now. Although, knowing David, he probably knew all along and will have a little chuckle if he reads this. So I guess he is having the last laugh. Nevertheless, he is a lovely guy and I hope he found a special lady and was blessed with children.

Chapter 6

No Business Like New Business

It was April 2002 when I was awarded *Maxim's* International Woman of the Year for the third time. The event was pretty spectacular and a lot of fun. Pictures taken on the red carpet that year show me in a short, pale-blue dress with bell sleeves, and I'm looking confident and happy. My life was great but looming on the horizon was the big 3-0. Yes, I was to be 30 in October of that year and whilst to most people this would pass by in a blaze of partying, surrounded by good friends, to me it signified an ending of sorts.

By this point I'd been on the cover of hundreds of magazines from *GQ, Esquire, FHM* and *Loaded,* to women's magazines like *New Woman, Cosmopolitan* and *Vogue* and all kinds of other titles across the world. I was still travelling three or four times a month, still plugging away at those German catalogues, which literally made me millions.

I was a saver: I looked after my money or I invested it wisely, usually in property. I'd decided a few years before that I didn't want anyone else looking after my money; I would do it all myself. I was still traumatised by the memories of my mom losing all her money and of me struggling to pay the rent in New York and living on bagels.

I don't think that will ever leave me. I'll always be driven by a kind of fear around money, combined with an entrepreneurial spirit. Maybe that's the American in me: I've noticed that Brits are generally a little more embarrassed about the fact they want to make money, but if money buys you independence then I think it brings you confidence, too. This is what I've discovered over the years and is what I tell people when I do my business talks to 'mumpreneur' groups and businesses.

I was always aware that to last ten years as a model is unusual; to last into your thirties is pretty unheard of, unless the process of reinvention really comes off. There aren't many examples around of models who stay in the public eye once they've been through the peak of their careers. Yes, the supermodels like Kate Moss, Naomi Campbell, Christy Turlington and Cindy Crawford are still securing campaigns, but these women are brands in themselves and are still very powerful today. Charlize Theron, the South African supermodel had worked as an actress alongside her modelling career for a long time, and would go on to win an Oscar for *Monster*, where she played a serial killer. Elle Macpherson, too, had expanded her career into acting and presenting.

I had made it my business to stay relevant by working in TV as much as I could; I'd had a go at launching a music career but this had stalled when my second single, 'Once Around the Sun', reached number 24. It was a great song and I was really proud of what I'd done but clearly, the music had been a grounding for other things.

I was as busy as ever with photo shoots and TV offers but I could see a time when this might all come to an end or, at least, tail off. And I wanted to know that I was ahead of the curve and that I wouldn't have nothing else in my life but modelling. Jobs I'd got along the way brought in a lot of money – like the Pot Noodle TV ad in 2002 (in one shot I had to wear a bald wig!) and the Diet Coke ad in 2003 where I was shown careering off in a forklift truck! – but I needed something I could own and grow.

I was already plotting an exciting next step. I had no idea then that the idea would take my life in such a different direction, the end result of which would result in a business that now brings in seven digits.

I'd been toying with various ideas for some time and I was looking for a product I could endorse that I felt tapped into the essence of the Caprice 'brand' and, most importantly, gave something useful to women.

Meanwhile, a man called Terry Green had dramatically changed the fortunes of the department store Debenhams. He had brought in high street 'diffusion' ranges created by established designers. The shops had gone from being dowdy and old-fashioned into glamorous, modern department stores. He said at the time he wanted it to feel like coming into Debenhams was like 'walking into a glossy magazine'.

Terry is a self-made millionaire with bags of energy and enthusiasm and a great understanding of retail, and so it was to him I decided to take my idea – which was to create a lingerie brand using my name and photographs of me, and promote it exclusively in Debenhams.

At that time, it was very unusual for a celebrity to endorse a brand new range in this way. It was a crazy idea of mine and I had no idea how to do it but I just knew it had legs.

I knew I'd have some sweet-talking to do. I mean, who was I? Just some model who flitted around going from one party to the next – why should he take me seriously?

My agent was with me on this though. We both had a gut instinct that we were onto something and he did the legwork, calling Terry a number of times to set up the meeting. When we finally made it into the head office in Marylebone, London, I was thoroughly prepared.

'Terry, I think your lingerie could do with an injection of glamour,' I told him, cheekily. Remember, this is a man who knows retail like the back of his hand and I was bringing something new to him – he wasn't going to be easily persuaded. It's ironic that nowadays everyone is used to celebrities fronting the product ranges. So I told him I could create the awareness through millions of pounds-worth of marketing and through this, drive sales. Not only with my lingerie brand but through his entire store. At that time my mug was in at least one national newspaper a day – now, that is power, and I wasn't utilising it. I convinced him: yes, this is a big investment and there is an element of risk because it's never been done before, but I want you to think about it. It's going to work.

I can understand why he took some persuading now. As someone with my own business, I get that it's extremely tough to launch a new brand. Not only that, licensing was pretty untested back then and maybe he felt Debenhams were being used as a guinea pig. But thankfully, Terry hasn't become successful by being cautious and, thankfully, he took on my idea and ran with it.

We signed a contract and from signing on the dotted line to getting the products into stores took about six months. Either of us could get out of the contract whenever we wanted as there was a series of 'break clauses' written in there.

The collection was designed, produced and sold by the Debenhams team and, beyond using my image, I wasn't involved at all. We put out a range with balcony and plunge bras, low-rise thongs, and some very pretty (and very sexy) basques. The first season, sales were phenomenal. Terry was the flavour of the moment and it was well deserved.

As a result of the success of the range, Debenhams decided to use me in a pre-Christmas TV campaign for the store. I was so pleased: they were willing to invest a lot of money (TV campaigns cost millions) to promote my range and so there was a lot riding on the sales' success.

It was such a fun shoot – I spent the day rolling around in a bed, supposedly naked (the truth? I had my knickers on!) and pretending to search my bedroom high and low for my lingerie.

I had to look at the camera and ask, 'Have you seen my lingerie?' before the camera cut to images of Debenhams and back to me saying, 'Found it!'

It was great! The campaign was showing everywhere in the Christmas run-up, a key time for stores to sell lingerie, and I waited to see what would happen with the sales figures. I had everything crossed because as part of the licensing agreement I would get a percentage of the sales, on top of a signing-on fee with Debenhams.

I'll never forget walking into the store for the first time, I think it was the one on Oxford Street in London, to see a relatively small section promoting the range. I've gotta say, I looked great! There were pictures of me modelling the lingerie, as well as my signature in bright pink, and the range, which was lots of bright colours, really stood out.

Debenhams had spent a fortune though and of course I wanted sales to continue to soar – a win–win situation for both of us. But I needn't have worried because that range sold out! Bear in mind at this time I was at the height of my fame and in the newspapers every day. This profile, combined with the TV ad and the fantastic work the Debenhams team had done, made it all work like a dream and for the next five years, my lingerie was a huge success story for them.

As time went by Debenhams estimated about two million women were wearing something from my range. I was dubbed 'Queen of the Undieworld' by the press and I loved it – it's a moniker that has followed me around ever since and I'm not complaining!

Whilst my lingerie range (and me wearing it) was being plastered over billboards, I continued to work hard with magazine shoots, catalogues and TV.

But the real biggie for me that year was hosting an evening at the Oscars. I had to do live feeds for the TV network ABC, which was all pretty terrifying because there were so many factors that could go wrong. I remember being up on a terrace above the red carpet as everyone arrived. I had a brilliant view of the celebrities and had to talk about everyone as they walked in – so I did a lot of research beforehand.

'Here comes Jada Pinkett and Will Smith and every time they go out to a big event, Jada picks out what Will is wearing. And they might have a little bit of an argument about it but, usually, he ends up wearing what she wants him to wear…'

I had no one feeding me the information and so it really was a question of winging it, as they say in the business, so it was a good job I'd done my research. I also did a live feed from the after-show party on the same night. I was with a comedian and a famous stylist and we had to really dish the dirt. It was the year Gwyneth Paltrow wore that black and nude cream dress and we really went to town on her! It was my 'Joan Rivers' moment – fun but very scary, I don't know how people do that job on a daily basis.

Off the back of the Oscars, I was also asked to present behind-the-scenes at the American Music Awards (AMAs) and to present an award. I remember being introduced to the audience by Jon Bon Jovi as 'The most beautiful woman he'd ever seen'. I couldn't believe it! Bon Jovi were megastars and everyone had a crush on Jon. I was very, very flattered! Those years were just non-stop *wow* for me.

But even though I knew I was at the top of my game, as I've said, I knew this wasn't going to last forever. When you're young, you think that you know what you want and where you're going and that you're pretty much invincible – and that somehow you're in control of your destiny. I'd now had a lot of time in front of the camera and time on stage promoting my music but I was getting bored with the modelling.

By now, I could do it standing on my head and I wanted to try something new.

I'd had some experience of acting and I'd been cast in a couple of movies with Penélope Cruz, Vinnie Jones and the late Brad Bentro. By the time I hit my late twenties I realised I wasn't exactly Meryl Streep but I had been bitten by the bug. I wanted to learn more and where better to do this than by acting on stage and learning something about the craft involved?

The Vagina Monologues is a stage play, which uses three actresses to portray different aspects of being a woman, and it covers some fairly controversial topics like rape, female genital mutilation and masturbation. I'd seen the play and I loved it because it's so direct and yet it manages to be funny and empowering for women, all at the same time.

I wanted to do this play, very much. But I was nervous: how would I be received? Would anyone take me seriously as a credible actress? My agent contacted a man called Mark Goucher, who is an incredibly talented and prolific theatre producer and now has a zillion hits to his name. Mark was not keen to have me on board. 'No one thinks of Caprice as an actress,' he said, damningly.

But my agent persisted and sent over a show reel from various projects I'd been involved with over the years, and Mark agreed to audition me. After the reading, I felt so nervous because this was such a new direction for me and I wanted to be good at the job and accepted by the industry. I knew they were reluctant to cast me but that 'fuck you, I'm going for it anyway' attitude has always stood me in good stead and again it paid off! I got the part and I was delighted.

I was scared to death. Anyone who's worked in live theatre knows there are so many things that can go wrong and this was my first experience of doing a run in live theatre in the West End.

The play was to run at the Arts Theatre and I was cast with comedians Helen Lederer and Gina Yashere. I was well aware that these two were seasoned actors and I was the rookie but, somehow, I managed to pull it off with their help. The reviewers were very kind to me and the tabloid wrote:

'The evening's most pleasant surprise is supermodel and all-round celebrity Caprice, who demonstrates a lively and engaging stage presence, her almost alien beauty working extremely well in relation to the earthy, bawdy tone of the night.' Pretty good!

I did have one slightly embarrassing moment, however. I was invited onto the ITV show *This Morning* presented then by Fern Britton and John Leslie. Obviously I was there to talk about the play and about my role in it but I sort of forgot about the fact that it was the middle of the morning, a very long way before the 9pm watershed.

'So, what kind of monologues are you doing as part of the show?' John asked and I blithely told them: 'One of them is called Reclaiming Cunts'. The two presenters were utterly professional and moved on without blinking an eye. I didn't even think about it until later, when they told me what I'd said and two viewers complained. Apparently the complaint was upheld but it could have been so much worse. It seems my American accent had served me well; most people hadn't heard what I'd actually said on live TV!

The play had whetted my appetite for theatre and I was desperate to try another project, and learn as much as I could. The Broadway hit musical *Rent* was coming to the West End later that year and was being produced by none other than Mark Goucher again. I told my agent I wanted to do *Rent* and she said, 'Are you joking? It's a huge show, are you sure you're up to it?' But I was determined. I called up Mark and he said, 'Cap, there's no way you're experienced enough for this.' I thought, 'What? So I can't even audition for the part? This isn't right.'

And so I decided to get my tush down there and line up with everyone else on what's called in the business an 'open call' – where basically anyone can turn up. I waited in line with all the other actors. I was signing autographs and posing for pictures whilst I stood outside in the queue. It was slightly bizarre. I went into the studio for the audition and sang my heart out and I must have impressed them enough because a few days later I got the call. I was in! I was to play the part of Maureen, a lesbian performance artist.

I had to kiss another girl on stage as part of my role but I'd been in front of the cameras for years so it didn't faze me at all, although I found the singing tough on my voice. This was when I realised that years of training are needed when you're doing a big show like this because your voice has to be tough enough to stand up to the strain of singing every night. The rest of the cast were great – they could have been hard on me turning up there as a celeb and getting a part but I think they knew how hard I'd worked to get in and how much I wanted it. We all became really close during the run, which opened at the Prince of Wales Theatre on 15th December 2002.

In the meantime, I'd turned down a show called *Celebrity Big Brother* to be in the play, but I'd get another chance at Big Brother a few years down the line…

The following year I saw a show called *Debbie Does Dallas: the Musical* at a theatre in Oxford and I loved it. You might have heard of it because in the seventies it was something of a porn classic but the stage show is actually about a bunch of cheerleaders trying to make something of their lives. So, obviously, this had some resonance for me!

I spoke to Mark Goucher about bringing it to the West End and told him I wanted to play the lead, but the timing wasn't right. I didn't want to let it slip through my fingers though; I had high hopes for the show: I felt it had legs but it just needed tweaking. And so I decided to do something a little bit crazy – I took off to New York and bought the rights from the owners and said, 'Give me a year, I'm going to put this musical on.'

I wanted to workshop the show before I brought it to the West End. This way I could work out all the kinks and sort out the rewrites. I needed somewhere with access to great actors that wasn't going to cost a fortune; it would need to be cheaper than London. At the time I had launched my brand By Caprice into South Africa's big retail chain Edgars. I was already spending a lot of time there so I thought I could source investors and put on a short run of *Debbie Does Dallas: the Musical* on in Johannesburg.

I was to play Lisa, the school slut. And, no, it most certainly wasn't typecasting – remember, I never had a one night stand! The new script was written by my friend Kelly Marcel, who's a great comedy writer and has since written the screenplay for *Saving Mr. Banks* starring Tom Hanks and Emma Thompson. She's so talented. The play was fantastic and we had great reviews. High on its success, we were all geared up to bring the musical to the UK – when the bottom fell out of the economy worldwide.

Suddenly, just breaking even was the most important thing for me. I had spent a lot of money putting on the show, even with other investors; in the end we did just about make the money back but it was very tight. It made me nervous and after some consideration, I decided then wasn't the time to bring 'Debbie' to the West End. I'd love to do it one of these days though; it's a great show and such fun. Since then I have acted again a few times and I was in a movie called *Perfect Woman* in 2004, another with Vinnie Jones in 2006 and I was also in a movie called called *Hollywood Flies*. I've acted in TV series too (*Hollyoaks, After Hours*) which was fun, but these days, I think my talents are more of the entrepreneurial kind.

I'd managed to avoid my 30th. I really did pretend it wasn't there: I metaphorically stuck my head under the duvet, kept myself busy and quietly mourned the loss of my 'youth' as I saw it. It couldn't have been more different from my 40th birthday, which I celebrated with a huge party thrown for me by my partner Ty. For me, my 30th was something I just wanted to completely avoid altogether.

I didn't feel ready to settle down with anyone either. I was having too much fun, although it would irritate me to read one week that I was going out with Prince Albert of Monaco (we'd sat next to each other at an awards do, for heaven's sake, that's all!), Lee Ryan of boy band Blue (are you joking?

Lee's absolutely gorgeous and we're friends, but that's it) or 'serial loverboy', Callum Best (this is because I spoke to him once at a GQ awards do and suddenly we were supposedly an item).

In fact, I was much more likely to have been dating men who weren't in the public eye, but no one ever wants to hear about the non-famous guys. Not about the fireman – my god, he was hot – nor the Mr Normals. I dated some great guys. And some not so great. Anyway, the way I see it, each of those men I dated was just helping me learn about what I really wanted in a man and, thankfully, I found him. But that's a story for later in the book.

I continued with my various entrepreneurial projects. Up until the financial crash in 2008, I would buy homes in distressed situations, for example if the couple selling it were in the middle of a divorce or they'd run out of money and needed to get out of the house quickly – sometimes the houses had been repossessed by the bank. I would do them up and flip them (sell them on).

Florida, for me, was something of a gold mine at this stage. The area where Tiger Woods lived was obviously very affluent and I would buy property as they began the build, right at the early stages. I'd put, say, the ten per cent deposit down and by the time the house was finished, I'd buy it outright, hold it for two years in order to avoid capital gains and then sell. I owned three other properties internationally as part of my property portfolio.

I also landed a fantastic campaign for Paradise Poker, who paid me seven figures to promote poker over the next few years. They must have heard that I wasn't just a pretty blonde

– I was a blonde who knew how to swim with the sharks! Remember, I'd played poker for years with my family, during those fun Friday night dinners as a kid. I was something of an expert – or just really lucky. Actually, probably the latter. I loved poker and so, for me, it wasn't a hardship to have to go to Vegas to play a game of poker at the World Series, which is what they wanted me to do.

Over the next year I made appearances for Paradise Poker at all kinds of high profile events around the world and there are still YouTube clips of me explaining how to master the basics of the game. It might not have been an expected route for me to go down but it paid well and I felt very comfortable in that world – confident in what had always been a very male environment.

It seemed this was a deal that worked for everyone involved. In the first year I was working with the company, they were the seventh-highest performing gambling company in the UK and, by the time this campaign was over, they were number one. The company were so pleased, they asked me to do another year – happy days all round!

Towards the end of 2004 I was asked to appear on *Celebrity Big Brother*. This was the third celebrity version of the show and it was just huge. The show was pulling in 12m viewers and I was a big fan anyway. In terms of viewing figures and credibility, nothing beats the Oscars or the AMAs, but in terms of profile, in the UK, nothing came close to *Celebrity Big Brother*. I'd have been mad to turn it down and, anyway, I had experience of reality shows. I could hold my own – at least, I thought so.

Actually, I wasn't quite as prepared for the experience as

I'd first thought. The incredible mix of people in there was a recipe for drama, and early on the famous feminist and writer Germaine Greer walked out. She hated the whole experience and left after telling us she felt we were being bullied by Big Brother.

Other contestants were also pretty… interesting. Brigitte Nielsen was a total pro at reality shows; it was how she was making her money at the time. I liked her during the show but after the show she was a completely different person, and wouldn't acknowledge anyone. Big Brother made what some thought of as a genius move – others looked on with horror – in bringing in Jackie Stallone, Brigitte's ex-mother-in-law. The two of them had famously had a very difficult relationship and so of course sparks flew. It made compelling viewing and the series went down as one of the highest ratings for *Celebrity Big Brother*.

I really felt for Brigitte. It's everyone's worst nightmare but I think she's a tough cookie and she handled it well most of the time. They even appeared to smooth over some of their issues by being thrust together in the house for so long.

I detested one of my fellow housemates though, the horse-racing pundit John McCririck. He was an awful man. He and I rowed over the fact he said I'd had an easy life because I was good looking, going on to say: 'No, the best thing is for men to go out with ugly girls because they're grateful for what they get,' which obviously caused an outcry in and out of the house. For some reason his wife didn't take offence at this kind of statement. It's beyond belief that any woman would put up with a bigot like that in a marriage but, hey, each to their own I guess.

John would incessantly fart and pick his nose. He would fart all through the night and he really smelled disgusting, but worse than that were his horrible sexist views of women. I suppose he achieved what he'd set out to do: gain as much press exposure for himself as quickly as possible. And it did put him in front of an audience who'd never heard of him before.

Yes, there were some big egos in that house and the result was, I kind of went in on myself. I discovered I wasn't actually interested in grabbing as much air time as possible, I just wanted to protect myself. I didn't talk very much; all I had to do was put on a bikini a few times and the producers were happy!

There were some hilarious moments though. I remember having to pluck pheasants in a medieval lady's costume and I also had to dress up as a pig. It was all pretty ridiculous but it made great TV. I became really close to the DJ Lisa I'anson in the house and we're still good friends now. The actor Jeremy Edwards and I got on very well too; we're still friends. The two of us came out of the house together on day 16, two days before the final, so I was pretty happy with that, especially as my being in there raised £30,000 for Childline, my nominated charity for the show. The only thing I was not happy about was walking out on that chilly evening to see a waiting Davina and no boyfriend. The man I was seeing at the time had decided he didn't need to come and meet me. Big mistake – he didn't last long after that.

When you've been shut away like that for over two weeks, without being able to fully relax and without having people you love nearby, it really sucked to see nobody waiting for me. Davina handed me the phone and they'd got my mom on the line, which immediately made me burst into tears!

My mom and I talk almost every day, always have done, and so it had been extremely difficult not hearing her voice for all that time.

The day after leaving the show, I took my dogs for a walk on the heath near where I lived and it was absolutely nuts. All these dog walkers were coming up and asking for my autograph and there were paparazzi photographers everywhere. I had no idea that the show would have such a massive following but people loved it so much back then.

For weeks afterwards I was virtually mobbed in the streets – I remember once being in the back of a taxi and talking to a friend on the phone when I heard a click. I asked the driver what the noise was because I was getting suspicious; he was taking a little too much interest in me. I demanded he lift up the newspaper he had on his lap, only to see he had been recording my entire conversation. I could not believe it! I don't mind people being upfront about what they are doing – if you want to take a picture, fine, I understand that it comes with the fame territory but recording my conversation without my knowledge is not OK.

Another by-product of *Celebrity Big Brother* was the surge in the sales of my Caprice lingerie range in Debenhams. That season's range pretty much sold out – appearing in my bikini must have done the trick! This got me thinking. I knew the business was strong and I also knew my time at the top would not be everlasting. Debenhams would eventually drop me for another popular face of the moment. So I thought I should terminate my licence deal and supply lingerie myself. I would call it By Caprice lingerie and I would not be limited to one stockist. My distribution could be everywhere, including internationally. It would put me in control of my professional destiny and not vulnerable to anyone replacing me. However, I did retain my licence deals for a range of hair products – hair dryers, ceramic hair straighteners – which were selling well through various outlets. For me, it was all about exploiting my personal brand. Everyone knew my name and I wanted to use this in any way I could. Maybe, just maybe, I could manufacture and market my own brand from scratch, taking the whole profit and not just a cut.

I'd been careful with my money. I had regular income coming in on the sales of calendars, campaigns and TV work and the hair range as well as good property investments in America and the UK. I wanted to use that money to fund this project, rather than going to an outside investor, which is often what people do when they need to raise capital.

I thought, 'I can do this myself, how can I fail?' Mmm. Sometimes that over-confident American streak can trip a girl up! I do believe that the entrepreneurial spirit in me couldn't have held my ideas down for long though. I needed to prove to myself I could do it and in 2006, using £263,000 of my own money, I bought the licence back from Debenhams. This meant I was free to market my own lingerie line, although I kept up a good relationship with Debenhams and I stocked my line exclusively with them for the first season only. I had a lot to thank them for.

But before By Caprice could really get into its stride, something happened that would knock all thoughts of expansion out of my mind for a while.

Chapter 7

The Day the Wheels Came Off

All the way through the majority of my twenties, I'd steered clear of alcohol because I hated feeling out of control and, apart from anything else, it was unprofessional to turn up hungover on a job if someone was paying you – and why would I risk a deal with a company like Debenhams because of my lack of self-control? I've always prided myself on being professional and I felt if I drank, I'd be opening up all kinds of behaviour, which I could end up regretting.

Drugs back then, especially cocaine, were easily accessible and it didn't bother me if people wanted to take them – 'go on, snort yourself to death, knock yourself out…' I wasn't judgemental about it but it just wasn't something I was interested in. What was annoying was the queue for the ladies loo at the nightclubs. Everyone was in there taking drugs in the cubicles – and I just wanted to pee! I'd usually end up running into the men's instead, much quicker that way…

The only experience I'd had with drugs (apart from the mushrooms in New York) was completely accidental and happened when I was dating a guy in LA, around the time I met Prince Andrew. I'd been staying with him and I woke up one morning with terrible period pain. I asked him if he had any painkillers. And he told me where the Tylenol was in his bathroom. I popped a couple of them and got ready to go to my spin class at the gym.

This guy called Andy came to pick me up to go to the class and I got there and started to do my spinning. I sat on the spinning bike and… I was spinning… and I was spinning… and I was spinning until all of a sudden I fell off the bike. I was flat out on the floor but my legs carried on spinning and spinning into the air. At the same time I was trying to talk but I was just kind of making this weird grunting noise. I didn't know what the hell was going on.

Andy called my boyfriend and said: 'There's something wrong with your chick, she just fell off the spinning machine and she's lying there like a loon. Everyone thinks she's lost it, she's lying on the floor spinning her legs and making this weird noise.'

The boyfriend immediately knew what had happened. 'Oh shit, I told her to go to the bathroom to get the Tylenol but I think she's taken pills from the aspirin bottle where I keep my Quaaludes. You'd better bring her home to get over it.'

Quaaludes are now illegal in the US but for years they'd been used by people going out clubbing because they are a muscle relaxant. The boyfriend did freak out a bit because an overdose can be really dangerous. But as it turned out, one of the other side effects of the drug is that it increases sexual arousal, so once the worst of the drowsiness had worn off, he was quite happy I'd accidentally taken them…

Of course there's no way I'd go back to that gym. I'm not holier-than-thou about drugs, I just have a really bad reaction to them and I hate the way you can't control how long the effects will last. With alcohol I can make it stop by eating some bread or drinking water but with drugs it just doesn't work like that.

So even in the craziness of partying in London, I'd stick to the odd glass of champagne or a vodka. Then out of the blue one evening at some entertainment party or other I had a few more than usual and I thought, this is fun, and that was it. I guess I'd relaxed after almost 15 years in the business and decided to cut myself a little slack.

The time it all went wrong was in the run-up to Christmas 2005. As usual at this time of year, there was a lot of socialising, parties and people to see. I was spending the evening with my friend Kelly Marcel, who I'd worked with on the *Debbie Does Dallas* script. I picked her up in my black sports-class Mercedes and we drove into the West End. I parked in the Soho car park and we headed to Soho House, a private members club that attracts a lot of people in the entertainment business.

Kelly and I were having a great time and as the evening wore on, a few guys and various people we knew joined us. Soho House is the kind of place where people passing your table just join you for a drink and the evening goes on and on. Everyone was in a lovely, festive mood, and I was drinking and laughing away and probably didn't eat very much.

As I didn't normally drink to excess I always knew I could drive. But tonight I'd let go. Stupid. Beyond stupid.

At about 3am, the club kicked us out and we headed back to the car park to drive home. Kelly was going to come and stay at my house in north London and so we began by driving up Tottenham Court Road. She decided she wanted to head back to her house and not spend the night after all, so she asked me to pull over in a layby so she could hail a cab home.

As I was leaning over to kiss her goodbye, I noticed some cops walking over and eyeing me suspiciously.

I wound down the window and said the automatic: 'Do you want my driver's licence?' which is what the cops in America always ask to see. He just stared into my eyes and asked: 'Have you been drinking?' There was no way I was going to lie about this, I probably stunk like a drunken skunk anyway. 'Yes,' I admitted and immediately he asked me to get out of the car so I could be breathalysed. It turned out that I was just over the legal limit.

It's been reported that I used the phrase, 'Don't you know who I am?' – I honestly can't remember, but I wouldn't be surprised if I did. As I've said, at this point my ego was pretty rampant, the cops were being very mean and I was feeling very defensive and embarrassed. It's no excuse for saying something so butt-clenchingly awful but, in my defence, no one knows how they'll behave in the middle of being interrogated by the police.

That was it. I was arrested on the spot and put into the police van. Thank god Kelly was still with me, I'll be eternally grateful to her for sticking around through the next couple of hours. I remember sitting in the van, staring into the distance and over and over again saying to myself: 'How could you be so stupid, Cap?' I was so mad with myself for being so irresponsible.

We arrived at the station and I had to have my mug shot taken. It was so humiliating but one of the cops was very sweet: 'Don't worry, we'll breathalyse you again and see if your points have come down.

At 5am I was still just over the limit and so all the paperwork had to be filled in whilst I was waiting. For some reason they were very mean to Kelly, who by this time was hungry and tired. They wouldn't let her leave the waiting room, even though she wasn't being charged with anything. I was fortunate enough to not get slung into a cell; I was just left alone on a bench with my thoughts whilst I waited for everything to be completed.

When I was released in the morning the newspapers had already found out I'd been pulled over. How the hell did they get this information? I'd just been released from the police station. I guess you can draw your own conclusions. I climbed wearily into a cab, switched on my mobile phone and immediately saw a million messages from my manager.

'Cap, call me. What the hell has happened? My phone is blowing up!' I picked up one message after another from my agent, all saying the same thing. Everything went crazy; all the papers and magazines wanted to know the story. I don't remember giving any interviews at this time because all I wanted to do was crawl under a stone and die. I couldn't even call my mom, I was too embarrassed to admit I'd been drinking and driving.

The one person I did call, on the advice of a friend, was so-called 'Mr Loophole': the lawyer Nick Freeman. Mr Freeman was famous as a celebrity defence lawyer who specialised in traffic offences. He'd been responsible for helping David Beckham demolish an eight-month driving ban and he'd persuaded the court to punish a driving offence with points on Frank Lampard's licence rather than an outright ban.

I wasn't sure what he could do for me but we spoke at some length and he asked me a lot of weird questions, most of which I couldn't understand the relevance of to my case. One of the questions was, 'Were you on any medication?' I had been on antibiotics for a bladder infection. I had cystitis, something I'd been suffering from on and off for years.

It certainly wasn't something I wanted broadcast in court but if he thought it would help in some way, I trusted him to run with it. I had to pay for a series of tests, which would show whether the medication had any effect on the amount of alcohol my body absorbed. Anyway, it was pretty silly I hired him in the first place as I lost the case. I was fined £3,500 and was banned from driving for 12 months plus it cost me £30,000. I should just have taken full responsibility for my negligent actions and called it a day.

The following August, I came out of the courthouse after the hearing and there in front of me were at least 50 paparazzi and film crews all pushing for a comment. I had said at the time: 'Hopefully people will learn from my regretful experience. Do not drink and drive. That's all I have to say.' I reflected on what I'd done and admitted to myself that I could have caused an accident – I could have killed someone – and I deserved all the punishment I got.

Of course, By Caprice had only recently launched and it was touch-and-go whether this would really damage my brand. I made up worst-case scenarios in my head all the time: this is it, I lose everything I've ever worked for now and it's all my fault. Asda had just taken By Caprice swimwear on board. It was a massive account and when the news of my driving under the influence hit, they said they weren't going to touch my range and that what I'd done was damaging to their brand image. Other stockists were sceptical and all said they were 'considering' whether or not to sign their next contracts with me.

The big campaigns and the catalogue modelling slowed down and as the year went by, I sank lower and lower into depression. My mom, of course, was very worried. She told me: 'This is a lesson learned; you have to move forward.' She's tough, my mom! But she was right. I deserved this. The universe was, I believe, teaching me a lesson: to stop with the diva nonsense.

But there came a sort of feeding frenzy over my demise. One report said I'd tried to commit suicide by taking a drug overdose and had been admitted to the Priory, a rehab clinic, alongside reality star Jade Goody.

The Priory story was a step too far – in actual fact I was on a plane on the way back from South Africa where I'd been working on *Debbie Does Dallas: the Musical* at the very moment I was being identified as this person entering the clinic. I had my lawyers get involved and that national newspaper had to write an apology. I also went on *This Morning* to show the viewers my plane ticket to prove I had been on a plane and not in the Priory.

If anything confirmed to me that plans B, C and D are needed in life, this was it. But I am my mother's child – I was not about to be defeated. Even so, it took a while to build my confidence back up. My mom has always been a role model to me but I wasn't prepared to let depression wipe out the next ten years of my life in the way it had done her. I thought, 'Cap, you have to get out of this. Stay this way for the next decade? Forget it!'

Mom was partially instrumental in getting me back on my feet again. She'd call me every day and give me some of her tough love but really, I just got bored with feeling sorry for myself. I knew I had to roll up my sleeves and start that ball rolling again. I started to look at the cash flow for By Caprice: it was doing fantastically well, which meant I had the beginnings of a great business. I needed to build on that.

Chapter 8

Fighting Back

It was time for change. I had a word with myself: you're 35, you have to stop with all the young boyfriends. Hard for me to contemplate! They were just so hot – and there were never any headaches with them, they were fun and they had no major issues, just wanted to have a good time. But as time went by I began to think more seriously about what the future held and I had always had babies and children in the picture. It was so important to me. But marriage? Forget it. I don't need a piece of paper to validate my relationship in any case.

I met my new boyfriend, John, in the summer of 2007 in Ibiza when I was staying with my friends Laurence and Ivona. They have a beautiful house there and always invite lots of people for a holiday. John was a really nice guy who was ten years older than me and already had two children from a previous marriage. He was a 'proper' grown-up and very much in demand.

He had just broken up with Elle Macpherson and there were a lot of ladies after him. The first time I met him in Ibiza my friend and I had a bet: who would he go out with first? Of course I wasn't one to say no to an interesting bet! The next day, we went to James Blunt's house to hang out and John was there. We pretty much hit it off immediately and agreed to meet up later, and that was it: the rest is history.

John was very cool, he had his own business, he was funny and he had this artistic sensitivity that made him very attractive to me. I loved his vulnerability and he wasn't afraid to show it. I loved the fact that he was ten years older than me. I was finally in an appropriate relationship.

Before long we were talking about moving in together and I soon moved from my townhouse in Camden into his house in Notting Hill. We went out a lot to parties and events and we were a very social couple.

I've always considered myself quite a spiritual person and as I've said already, I'd come to realise that you can't really control your destiny. What you can do though is make the most of the life you have. For so many years I was sure about what I wanted, about the direction I needed to go in, and I worked hard to make my dreams come true. But as time went by, I began to pay more attention to 'signs' – without wanting to sound too hippy dippy about it, it's my belief that if you manage to calm your thoughts through meditation, great things happen. You have more clarity and tend to accept things as they are, not as you wish them to be.

I believe one should always have goals and desires but not obsess over them; let them go and it will happen when it's supposed to happen, not when you demand it. And you know what? It's nice to not think of five million things at once and to relax, even if it's just for 40 minutes a day.

Although I'd been meditating for a few years by this point, I was just self-taught. But when I lived with John I was introduced to a group of women who were regularly practising meditation together. They were such a lovely, special group of people and the lady who hosted the group took us through the technique every week. It took a long time to master: as anyone with a busy life knows, your brain is usually going 1,000 miles an hour with to-do lists or worries you find hard to put aside. Once you learn how to do it, I swear, it makes a big difference. I don't understand how it works, but it does work and I use it every day, even if it's just for a few minutes.

I had started to change my life. I was eating better, my stress levels had dropped through meditation, and I was sleeping like a baby, but I was still utterly exhausted to the point where I had a hard time getting out of bed.

'I've had it,' I told John one day. 'I have to find out what's going on with my body because this is just not me.' I'd always been very energetic and really strong and healthy and so I knew there had to be more to it.

When you're a model the pressure to look good and stay fit and healthy is immense, and eventually it kind of gets built into your DNA that you need to work at looking good in the same way anyone keeps their skills up-to-date in their job. Sometimes, the pressure to look perfect all the time and to have a rocking body really gets to you; it can batter your self-esteem to constantly feel you have to live up to a certain ideal. But I knew this came with the territory – at least ten years ago there was a little bit of room for 'reality' in photo shoots. Now, almost every last freckle is eliminated from photographs and it's such a shame.

I wasn't working out every day but I had a trainer at the gym and I had a running machine at home, so I was fit. I'd been a fish-eating vegetarian for years and was probably lighter in weight as a result. I'd been eating like this since my teen years, and it had always helped me maintain my weight.

I ate a strict veggie diet and took a whole host of supplements because I've always been someone who, if she looks at food, gets fat. It's in my genes! My mom always says, 'We have fat genes' and it's true, my family are not skinny particularly when we enter our thirtie's! Every now and then I still love to eat a double cheese and jalapeño pizza but apart from that, I'm still super-strict with my diet. I was never one of those models who'd say, 'I eat McDonalds all the time but I never put on any weight.' That was never me, I watched my food intake. Also, I was transformed by documentaries about the American meat industry. It's appalling how farmers treat these poor animals. Every time you take a bite out of a piece of meat or poultry, you're eating all the hormones that these monsters have put into the meat. I don't think I will ever be a meat-eater again as a result. Anyway, there's plenty of protein in tofu, beans and pulses. Meat just isn't for me.

A friend told me about a clinic in Surrey with a highly recommended naturopath who is also a qualified doctor. She's a wonderful lady who prefers to remain anonymous because she's inundated with patients, all of whom have come to her via personal recommendation. By the time I went to her I was virtually on my knees. This wonder-woman listened carefully to all my symptoms. 'You have to help me,' I pleaded. If she hadn't have been able to help, I'm not sure what I'd have done next.

She took about a million vials of blood from me and sent them off to the John Hopkins Hospital in Maryland, in the US, where they have a world-renowned biomedical research facility. I had to wait around ten days for the results and I was nervous because I'd never had anything seriously wrong with me before. Who knew what the hell was happening to me? There are so many horror stories around stress-related illness.

The results came back to reveal I had chronic fatigue syndrome (CFS), also known as ME – an unusual illness with a variety of causes and the symptoms described certainly matched some of mine: muscle soreness, a feeling of almost permanent exhaustion, especially after any exercise, frequent sore throat, interrupted sleep, and mood swings. In some ways it was a relief to know what the illness was, but I also realised after doing my own research that this was not a problem that was about to go away easily.

I read stories online of people who'd been ill for five, ten years, some of them completely bed-bound for long periods of time. I was terrified, I thought that this was just the beginning of the illness for me and I had to have faith in this clinician and her team that they would be able to help me before the illness really took a long-term hold.

There are still so many theories around the causes of CFS but typically it's thought it can start a while after some kind of virus has attacked your body, or hormonal problems, even allergies. In my case though, the doc believed it was related to the amount of mercury in my system. Mercury, as in the poisonous liquid metal, which used to be in our fillings? Yup, that kind of mercury.

Mercury is actually present in most fish in varying quantities and, because I've been a bit of a health nut for many years, I was eating tonnes of fish – especially tuna – which I ate virtually every day. It was my low-fat-but-high-protein meal of choice and had been for a long time. Unfortunately, tuna in particular seems to retain high levels of mercury and it can cause all kinds of problems, I've since learned. Too much tuna can lead to memory loss, heart disease, tremors and birth defects in babies born to moms who eat a lot of tuna. It was frightening to know that this was what was wrong and that I was gradually being poisoned in this way, especially when I'd prided myself on my healthy diet.

Naturally I was horrified. Hearing that your body is gradually being poisoned, that it's affecting your long-term health and that it might also have implications for your unborn child was horrifying. I love the NHS but it did make me worry about all those people who don't have access to the kind of clinic I could afford. The doc told me that the longer this condition is allowed to continue, the longer it takes to fix.

She also found something else. 'For some reason,' the doctor told me, peering in puzzlement at my results, 'you appear to have a high concentration of nickel and mercury in your body – especially around your pancreas.' On a scale from one to ten I was almost a ten, there was so much of it in my body. At this, a chill went through me. I'd lost my grandmother on Dad's side and grandfather on Mom's side to pancreatic cancer. When I told the doc she looked mildly alarmed but seemed quite clear about my treatment.

It became really important to do something about that toxic build-up and in fact she later asked if she could use me as a case study for her research.

First of all, I had to change my diet – I could eat fish but not the kind high in mercury or nickel and certainly no canned fish or fruit. I could eat eggs and it was recommended I eat white meat but I couldn't bring myself to do it. And the low-nickel diet – don't eat brown or wholemeal products – contradicted the low-mercury diet – *do* eat brown or wholemeal products, plus nuts and pulses. It was so confusing!

In the end I used my common sense. It was really the mercury poisoning that was the main issue, and the treatment began immediately. Then I started on 31 vitamins a day and a treatment called Lipid Replacement Therapy (LRT), which is relatively new in this country but which works by fundamentally cleaning out your entire system and, in particular, helps to detoxify your liver. This happened every week for the next year and a half. I'd sit there on one of those white plastic picnic chairs, hooked up to a machine that was pumping the good stuff into me, leaving me plenty of time to think.

For the first time, I started to wonder if my long-held dream of having a family might encounter problems. I'd thought I was as fit as a fiddle yet here I was, with three bags of nutrients going into my veins.

And then I got bronchitis.

I'd been feeling like I'd been run over by a truck for a while and I'd been warned that the side effects of the LRT can make you feel worse before you get better. In fact it would take months before it made a difference, but this is normal.

Your body is trying to release all the built-up toxins, which years and years of stress, environment and bad eating have stored up. It's like the deepest cleanse your body could get but at first your body has to work extra hard to release all this crap, and as a result your immune system is vulnerable. I was being quite aggressive with the treatment to begin with as I wanted to feel better; I was desperate to feel better.

One morning I could barely move – I was sweating and had a very high temperature. I was continuously coughing up an obscene amount of mucus. I went to my GP and he warned me that if we didn't sort this out right away it'd turn into pneumonia and he prescribed some antibiotics. I took them for two days and felt worse. I was really worried so I called up the clinic where I was having LRT treatment and they told me to come in right away. As I walked into the office, they whisked me away to a private room where I wouldn't infect any other patients. They hooked me up to an intravenous drip, which pumped in a very high dosage of vitamin C and zinc into my body.

It worked like a dream. If I can give just one health tip to my friends and family it's to take vitamin C and zinc if you feel a cold coming on! Within two days I was virtually back to normal – even my GP couldn't believe it, he was gobsmacked.

It took a good nine months for me to start to feel normal again after I'd been diagnosed with CFS and mercury poisoning. And the fact that the doc had identified what she believed to be a genetic weakness for my body to process mercury, nickel and probably other toxins, meant that I dramatically changed what I ate and drank, permanently. I now eat a very limited amount of fish and my mercury and nickel levels are very much under control. I was spending £40,000 a year on these treatments and 31 vitamins a day but finally I was clean and healthy.

John and I were both very busy with our businesses and we spent a lot of time apart, but more than that, the magic just wasn't there any more. When we were together, we would row a lot. We were together for almost three years but somehow, about halfway through, I think we both realised that this relationship wasn't going to be forever. We liked each other, loved hanging out together but that spark wasn't really there – we were just too different.

I'd kept hold of my house in Surrey and in the end John and I split up over the phone. I had a removal company move all my stuff out of his place and back to my home while I was out of the country. It sounds so casual but at the time it was easier that way, and John and I had mutual respect for each other. In fact, I was the one who introduced him to his current wife! She's a lovely lady and they are absolutely perfect for each other so we both ended up in a good place.

Apart from anything else, I needed all my energy to focus on By Caprice, because things had gotten a little bit rocky during that time. The small matter of a worldwide financial crash...

Chapter 9

Crashing, not Burning

Whilst I hit a low in my personal life in 2006 that took a long while to climb out of, from a business point of view things were actually going really well. After a bumpy start, I was getting the lingerie range right and increasing my stockists.

But it hadn't been easy. For starters, I almost wrecked the launch range, which was still being stocked by Debenhams, because I got it totally wrong. I overlooked the fact that Debenhams knew their market, knew what the customers wanted and had the wherewithal to sell it brilliantly. I was confident I knew what I was doing – after all, I knew customers loved the push-up bras and the young, sexy cuts, but I neglected the fit.

I naively thought the factory would do all the fit so when the samples arrived at my office for me to approve, I didn't have a technician check them over. Instead I just approved them all. When I sent Debenhams the gold seal – this is a term used for a sample from production – they quickly rejected the entire collection because the fits were so appalling. I almost lost my business in the first season. It was a lesson I will never forget. Thank goodness I had liquidity from my modelling career to fall back on.

I could almost see the £263,000 investment I'd put in to launch By Caprice, all of which was my own money, disappearing down the plughole. I had to be agile; I had to act fast and figure out how to put the pieces back together. I realised I had to get a technician, and learn every integral part about my trade. At the end of the day, I had to spend money on a team with the experience and education in retail behind them. I knew that meant spending more but ultimately, I'd make more money as a result. I also realised that the customer is not an impulsive buyer any more. You need to give them originality, quality and a competitive retail price. And most importantly, I realised that this was going to be a long battle and that I wasn't going to see a return in the next six months. I needed to have the passion to stick with this to make it really work.

You have to live and breathe your business and you've got to educate yourself thoroughly about your trade. And lastly, cash flow is key. I had to understand this. I knew what would be coming in and going out for the next nine months so if I could foresee a problem in the future I could react now to find a solution.

I called up Next and Shop Direct – who own Very and Littlewoods. They did take my call but at first that's as far as it went. I was Caprice the model, the stereotype that had haunted me for years. They were reluctant to invest as they thought I'd be here one day and gone a year later like all the other celebs. What they didn't realise was that this wasn't a licence deal any longer, I was the supplier! It took me a few years of stalking until finally I had great numbers and was making my presence known in the retail world as an entrepreneur and a successful brand.

Finally, Next and Shop Direct took By Caprice as one of their brands – wow, that day the team and I did a little dance around the office!

My first season with Next and Shop Direct was a huge success. Next had a replenishment order of almost 15,000 units per bra. That's when the reality dawned on me: how was I going to pay upfront for the bras to be made? This was a huge number, bigger than anything I was used to. The way it usually worked was that I'd have to pay my factories when the goods landed in the UK, then two months later I would finally get paid by my stockists.

I had money for the first round: I could pay for the manufacturing and the other costs involved, but beyond that I had no 'liquidity', which means I had no cash floating around to pay for them – without selling various properties to raise it. It was pretty galling. I was going to have to borrow some money from the bank. I mean who has over a million pounds in liquidity just hanging around in their bank account?

I hate asking anyone for money; it's just not in my nature. Especially when they're charging ridiculous fees in interest. But I had no other choice. And so I took myself off to Barclays to ask for a back-to-back temporary loan. They would front me the money and two months later I would pay them in full with interest, as that's when I'd be paid by my stockists.

My gorgeous balconette bras and thongs sold phenomenally well and it wasn't long before I was being stocked by online brands like ASOS and Figleaves as well as by the stores on the high street and in catalogues. It was a dream come true – but I couldn't relax yet. When a business is flying, that's the time to reinvent and this is what I did.

Not only did I have the stereotype to overcome but I was a woman in business. Perhaps it's a little different in the US – as a nation Americans are maybe more forthright and direct – but there's a general view even now that it's not polite or feminine to be 'pushy', and it annoys the hell out of me. We all have to make money, no matter what gender we are. If we need to behave like men to break that glass ceiling then hey, *c'est la vie*.

I signed another deal with Littlewoods that was more of a standard licence to model occasionwear for them. I started to build my own brand by launching By Caprice Swim in December 2007, and By Caprice Sleep in August 2008. The trademark look for all of my ranges is fun and fashionable to wear but with a sexier twist than similar ranges. I think I know what makes a woman feel good about herself and what she wears beneath her clothes or privately in her home should make her feel empowered and full of confidence.

I was still modelling all the garments myself at this point because I knew that my fame was my strongest marketing tool, but I was aware that at some point I'd need to use other models or 'names' to promote the brand. I couldn't go on modelling forever and anyway, using other faces and bodies was all part of developing By Caprice for new markets and the younger customers who might not know who I was.

I was particularly proud of the fact that my return rates were one of the lowest across the board with all my stockists. I took my 'fits' very seriously, especially because of the lesson learned with my first range. I had five models try on each garment because everyone's body is so different, and if my garments looked good on all five, we had a product ready for production.

I'd found three great factories in China to manufacture my products. My ambition was to go global. If you're going to do something, you might as well think as big as possible. I really felt I had my finger on the pulse because I was involved in everything from the modelling through to the design and finance.

I've always loved the design side of the business. I'm not a technician and I now had great people to deal with that side. In the meantime I discovered that I needed to go and look at the kind of fabrics coming through every season to make sure we were on top of the right colours, patterns and any innovations in materials.

And so I began visiting the fabric shows in Paris twice a year, which was a huge step for me because it meant I was staying ahead of the curve in design terms. The shows are great because you get to see future trends and source new trims, laces, embroideries.... It also meant I made a lot of contacts and would get a sense of what was going on in the markets. My ambition grew – I thought in terms of five-year plans and told my agent to turn down the *FHMs* and the *GQ*s. I needed absolute focus: I was no longer a model, I was a businesswoman who occasionally did some TV or the odd photo shoot, pure and simple.

I knew I needed to be much more careful about the image I portrayed to the media and I became selective about the photo shoots and the stories my customers or potential customers might read about me in the press.

My property portfolio was part of my security – it was there if I needed funding for the business as I could sell and use the money – until the financial crash in 2008. The economy fell and so did the value of all my houses.

I started to feel more than a little twitchy about the financial markets – if people weren't able to move, they couldn't take up new jobs or increase their wealth in any significant way. I know that for the average Joe or Jane, property is something, which once you own, you feel it will make you money somehow. If that stops happening then people lose their confidence.

And that is exactly what happened. Compulsive buying was dead. In other words people were thinking about what they were buying, wondering, 'Do I need this?': they were looking at the price point.

In fact, all buying was completely dead. When the giant American bank Lehman Brothers collapsed it started a domino effect. At first it looked like an isolated event and then, overnight, I lost over £1m. Just. Like. That. Actually it was more like £1.6m, which, for me, was an enormous amount of money.

This is the way it happened. I had to pay my factory owners in China in American dollars. Yet I would get paid by my stockists in sterling. Therefore I had learned to work the exchange market, which was very new to me. When I needed to exchange money, I would call my bank and ask them what the rate was. It was consistently two-to-one, which meant I would get $2m in exchange for £1m. Now that's a healthy return. However, I will never forget the day I called to ask for the exchange rate and it had nosedived from $2 to $1.37… I lost almost £1.67m overnight.

I'll never forget it. I felt completely and utterly sick; it was devastating. I lost so much money and what was worse, my stockists were all cutting their orders in half because no one was buying. The public had gone into shock over the news that the Northern Rock bank had collapsed and a series of other high street banks were to be shored up by the government. It's enough to make anyone scared of spending money they might not have and it finished off thousands of businesses. I freaked out completely – everything I'd ever worked for could turn to dust within months. I had to think very quickly about how to stem the decline.

There was absolutely no way I wanted any of my staff to be jobless – especially during a time when nobody was getting any jobs. I had five or six people, some with young families to take care of, on the books in the UK and there were the factories in China, which obviously I was creating contracts for and to see how concerned these people were was heartbreaking. I couldn't let them down.

The orders were being cut in half and I wasn't shifting the stock but I came out fighting: I knew I needed to change my business plan and so I had to find new factories and renegotiate my costs with every supplier I had. I flew backwards and forwards for weeks, going between China and London to sort everything out. I'd do 18 hours a day on these visits. It would kill me. Before the recession I'd had a middleman who sourced a lot of the materials on my behalf. Now I did this myself and not only did I save a 20 per cent margin but it also made the business more efficient.

I played hard-ball with everyone but I was very lucky in many ways because I had a stack of money I could fall back on from my modelling days and this is the key when you have your own business. Cash flow is *everything* – know it, understand it, learn it and live by it – it's your bible.

I didn't believe in having a financial advisor as I'd had a bad experience in the past. I kept on top of it all myself along with my bookkeeper and my accountant. Over the following months we rode that bumpy ride and it was so tough. I was so drained and scared but I knew there had to be solutions and I worked 24/7 to ensure I came through it with the business intact.

I became known for my frugality! I told an interviewer once I was living on £30 a week, which might have been a *slight* exaggeration but the sentiment is right – I've never splashed my money around but through this crisis I really battened down the hatches and was very conservative with my spending. My mom was a great advisor through this period as she'd gone through bankruptcy, and rebuilt a multi-million dollar business since then. I knew I had to look after my money and just keep the business going, as sooner or later economic conditions would improve. And they did. I kept all my staff and actually ended up employing more. We weren't just getting by, eventually we were thriving once again.

I launched the By Caprice bedding range and what I discovered was that even when the finances are stretched, women still want celebrity brands in their lives.

I realised long ago I need a goal to keep me interested, to keep me thriving, and it's not actually about making money. It's about having something that motivates me, that makes me get up in the morning and make something happen. I don't know if this is ambition or drive or whatever you call it but I have it, at least most of the time! I think, looking back on that time during the recession, I felt the most driven I've ever been because that survival instinct kicked in. The years I spent doing all the boring administration, learning about how the bookkeeping worked and being involved in every decision about my brand have so far paid off. I think it's the only way to work – learn the books, learn the fit, learn about profit and loss and future planning. If you have your own business, this is essential.

Chapter 10

Struggles – and Good Times

Whilst I was struggling along trying to salvage the business, I had a relationship with a very sweet guy called Juan, who was introduced to me via a friend at a dinner party. The only problem was that Juan lived in the Bahamas, which made our dating life a little tricky – or a little exciting, depending on which way you look at it! We went out with each other for a year and I'd go back and forth to his house over there. He set up an office for me in the house and I'd work from there most days but the voice in my head saying: 'Find the right man… get real, is this one special enough?' was getting louder and I had to pay attention! Juan was special, but not right for me.

I've often felt over the last ten years that each of the men I had any sort of 'proper' relationship with was sent to teach me something about what I did and didn't want from my man, and that sooner or later, those preferences would be whittled so finely, I'd immediately know when Mr Perfect appeared. Still, I'd started to get a little bit cynical about this, especially when my next fling was a man ten years younger than me. I was regressing!

I was introduced to a rugby player. But it was clear from the beginning that this was nothing more than a fling because he was so much younger than me. I'm sure he was thinking, 'What the hell am I doing?' in the same way I was! We went out with each other for about ten seconds but he was gorgeous, 6ft tall and built like a brick. I hadn't gone out with anyone like that before and I thought, OK, from now on, they gotta be tall!

It was a great fling but it just fizzled out. I don't think we were ever even photographed together. I honestly think I briefly regressed to my previous 'toy boy' dating pattern because my business was so tough at the time and I just didn't have the emotional capacity – or the time – to put into a 'grown-up' relationship. But, the L-word is no respector of time or international business commitments, as I was soon to find out.

Thankfully, business started to really pick up by the end of 2010 and at the back of my mind, I had another plan to investigate: using a model other than me to promote my ranges.

For me, this was huge. I knew from my research that when Elle Macpherson stopped modelling her own ranges, the sales figures had plummeted and it meant that I needed to do it very carefully if I was going to progress the brand, rather than damage it.

I couldn't go on modelling forever, well, not lingerie anyway. It wasn't going to work: my ranges are targeted at a fairly young market and the truth is, those girls want to see a model they can identify with in a lingerie campaign. Apart from anything else, it was boring having to still work out four or five times a week and eating like a rabbit! I'd had enough… No, I needed to move things on.

I still intended to appear in some of the campaigns, particularly swimwear, but I'd been thinking for some time about using a celebrity 'name' and as we played around with different ideas and types of girl, it became clear that our customers at the time were obsessed with a new show called *The Only Way is Essex* (*TOWIE*). This is, for anyone who hasn't seen it, a 'scripted' reality TV show, and it had really captured the public's imagination. In May 2011 it even won a BAFTA for its portrayal of a group of glamorous friends and their families in Essex.

One of the stars of the show, Amy Childs, was the real star. Amy was a beautician with a warmth and innocence that beguiled everyone who met her and she was soon being asked onto every TV chat show going. What I loved about Amy was her 'glam girl next door' aspect. I thought it fitted perfectly with By Caprice and if I was going to take a gamble by shooting my campaign with a celebrity, she was a good bet.

Amy arrived on set the day of our shoot in a little too much make-up, understandably – it was the look she was famous for. But I shut that look down, styled the shoot myself, hired the photographer, helped with the mood boards. I wanted to strip down her make-up and try to convince her to go for an entirely different look. I was scared to death to do this. I wasn't sure if she would break out into a stroppy diva tantrum act – something like I'd have done in the past. Let's face it, karma is a bitch; I'd have deserved it.

I presented various pictures of the kind of look I wanted for Amy but surprisingly, not only is she gorgeous, she's actually a really lovely person and she agreed. With no headaches.

When we got the pictures back they were so sweet. I think they're my favourites of all the celeb models we've used because she looks so fresh and gorgeous but also, the audience had a real affection for her and we got such a great response from everyone! I think the shots did really well for Amy as well as for By Caprice – everyone wanted them from the tabloids to magazines and websites. People were clamouring for them and sales went nuts.

I was too busy to put much time – or thought – to my love life. I was happy to keep things light but I knew I was ignoring the nagging voice telling me to get my act together and find the right guy.

'You have to meet this guy, his name is Ty Comfort, he's single and he's six years older than you.' My friend Ray, who works in the music industry, was on the phone trying to organise my love life for me. 'Hold on here, I'm currently dating a gorgeous man ten years younger than me and you want me to meet someone six years older?' I laughed. I was dating the rugby player but we both knew it was nothing serious and so I agreed, if the opportunity to meet this guy came up, I'd be open to it.

The opportunity arose sooner than expected. My friend Tara and I were heading over to Ultra music festival in Miami. It's a huge electronic music festival and we were in a sprawling tent filled with 30,000 people all dancing to a live set from Swedish House Mafia. There was a fantastic atmosphere as we made our way over to the VIP section where Ray was sitting with a group of people.

Ray said, 'Hey, Cap, this is the guy I've been wanting to introduce you to, Ty Comfort.' I looked over at Ty and thought, he's seriously hot. Ty is 6ft 4in with dark curly hair, hazel eyes, a perfect smile and body, and hands the size of England. Perfect!

I introduced myself. 'Hi, I'm Caprice, I've heard so much about you and it's great to meet you at last.' Nothing. Not a glimmer of recognition. Ty hardly even registered the fact I was standing in front of him, he just looked at me and looked back at the crowd in front of us.

'What a jerk,' I said to my friend Tara. 'Gorgeous, but a bit of a jerk.' And that was it, I thought no more about him because the night took off in a different direction and we weren't hanging out with the same people.

For a split second I thought, 'Oh god, have I lost it? I'm 39 and officially chopped liver.'

A few weeks later, back in the UK, Ray called me again and said, 'Let's all go to Shoreditch House and I'm going to bring Ty again.

I said, 'OK, but I'm not expecting anything. Let's face it, Miami was an epic fail.' But Ray was so insistent, he said Ty had drunk about a million vodkas the night I met him and I had to give him another shot.

That night I turned up at Shoreditch House, a private members club in east London, with the intention of seeing some friends and having a quiet drink. I had very low expectations of anything happening with Ty but when I walked in and saw him, I was shocked again at how much I fancied him! I pushed that to the back of my mind but this time we started talking and didn't stop for the next hour and a half.

We really did get on like a house on fire. Ty is also an American living in London, which might have given us some common ground, but it wasn't about that, there was a connection between us. I just felt really comfortable with him. I still thought he was utterly gorgeous but I had no idea what he thought of me.

Later that night, we all went to another party at some underground nightclub where my world-famous DJ friend Nic Fanciulli was playing. I got on the decks with Nic for a little while, which was fun, and when I'd finished I looked around, but no Ty. He'd gone. We didn't exchange numbers that night but I thought that, for sure, he would get my number from Ray and call me.

A day went by, a week, two weeks... OK, I thought, onto the next customer. I was very busy at work and I wasn't dwelling on Ty but it was weird because my instincts told me there was definitely something going on between us, but maybe I was wrong. Anyway, work was still very tough at this point and I was having to micromanage the business because the downturn in the economy meant that I couldn't take my eye off the ball at all.

I needed to fly over to LA on business in late June and I arranged to go and see my best friend Andrea Wynn in Vegas who I've known for the last twenty years. Andrea is married to the hotel magnate Steve Wynn, who owns incredible, palatial hotels the Wynn and Encore and he's famous for transforming Las Vegas with hotels like the Bellagio and The Mirage.

And so I was relaxing on Andrea's terrace, overlooking a beautiful golf course, catching up, when suddenly my phone rang. I didn't recognise the number but it was a private phone so I took the call. 'Hi Caprice, it's Ty. Ray told me you're in Los Angeles and I have to come out to LA for a meeting. I wanted to know if you'd like to go out for dinner?'

My ego, never very small, was also a little bit bruised. I said, 'I'm sorry, Ty, I'm not available right now, I'm with my girlfriend in Vegas.' 'OK, no worries,' he said and rang off. The second we got off the phone I wanted to hit myself. Why did I let my ego get in the way again? I berated myself: 'you know you wanted to see this guy, Cap, why are you playing these stupid games?'

Ten minutes later, my phone rang and it was Ty again. 'Cap, I'm on United Airlines flight blah blah blah from LA to Vegas and I'm going to take you out for dinner tonight in Vegas.' I was too stunned to speak, though I didn't say no!

After Ty hung up, I looked over at Andrea and said, 'Oh my god, this guy is a major player. He just told me he wants to take me out to dinner and he's flying out to meet me! This was one of the biggest player moves of all time. Andrea and I both started screaming and when we eventually came back to earth, she asked me Ty's surname.

She said, 'Oh my god, Cap, I've known this guy for twenty years! OK, I want to know everything, dish the dirt right now.' And that's when she revealed to me a little of Ty's past.

He'd only recently split up with his wife the previous year and he was going through the divorce. 'This is why you'd probably never met him before now,' she explained. Andrea went on to tell me what integrity he had. He had three children, he was a great dad and a thoroughly nice person.

Wow, a totally different picture from the one Ray had painted to me. He had told me that Ty was dating three gorgeous, 24-year-old models, had the most insane bachelor pad in Cadogan Square in the middle of London and was pretty much out every night but it didn't worry me too much. Newly divorced, we'd probably all do the same thing.

Most women would run for the hills but I, on the other hand, liked it because this was a challenge and I love a challenge.

Ty and I went out for dinner that first night with Steve and Andrea. The second we sat down for dinner, the interrogation began: Steve was very protective and only wanted the best for me. Some of the guys I'd gone for were totally wrong for me but hey, you have to kiss a lot of frogs before you find your prince.

Steve wanted to know it all, not from what I'd told them but straight from the horse's mouth: what Ty did for a living, what his situation was at home, with the family – Andrea hadn't seen him for years and it was the first time Steve had met him. Ty was as cool as a cucumber. He doesn't get intimidated; people find him intimidating usually but I didn't know that at this point. By the end of the night he had passed the test with flying colours. Steve was actually well impressed for the first time ever!

After dinner, Steve and Andrea wanted to give us a tour of their hotel and to show us XS, which is inside the Wynn

Hotel. XS is one of the top three grossing nightclubs in the world and you have never seen anything quite like it. It's opulent and beautiful with only the world's hottest DJs playing there. The design is said to be based on the curves of the human body, all of which helps to create just the right mood if you're on a first date with a gorgeous man.

So here we are walking through the nightclub and, oh my god, it's like the parting of the Red Sea! Everyone stood back as we came through. There were five security people on either side, thousands of gorgeous people in the club, but all eyes were definitely on us, which was great because I really wanted to impress Ty. You know what it's like on a first date – you want to look as hot as possible to impress, and I'm hoping I managed to do that!

After the club shut for the night at about 2am, we definitely weren't ready to call it a night. I took Ty to a strip club. Don't judge me – if you're in Vegas at that time of night, everyone goes to strip clubs because they are usually really great bars to hang out in, and I actually don't find them intimidating at all. As I walked in, I spotted a group of guys I hadn't seen in five years. I walked up, gave them huge hugs and started having a great gossip. After about ten minutes I noticed that Ty had disappeared and to this day, I have no idea where he went and nor do I want to know... but at this point in the relationship I think it's totally irrelevant. The important part is, I called him and he immediately answered the phone. I asked him if he was still in the club and I suggested we get the hell out of there.

He immediately said, 'I'll meet you at the front door,' and we jumped in a taxi and headed back to the hotel but we still weren't ready to call it a night. I suggested we hit the black-jack table and he said, 'Let's go!'

We sat down at the table and there was a couple sitting there from Michigan and they were on their honeymoon. They were so lovely and we sat and played blackjack with them for three hours. We had a few drinks and the mood was great, we were all so 'up'. The atmosphere was really exciting and there were no signs of anyone being ready for bed anytime soon. By then it was about 8am and we all thought, right this is getting a little bit sad, we need to go to sleep! We hugged the newly-weds, wished them luck with their future and headed towards the lift.

Ty asked me if I wanted to come up to his room. Now… I'm not playing the holier-than-thou card but you never accept an invitation to a man's room unless you want something to happen – and you know what I'm talking about.

A one night stand really isn't my thing. I love the chase, the butterflies, the tension and the teasing – now that is fun. And then finally getting to know that person and the build-up to the night you give in and have amazing passionate sex – that's what I'm talking about. But fuck all that, I went to his room anyway!

We walked in and sat on the sofa, talked for a bit and then he grabbed me and kissed me passionately. His hands started inching towards my breasts and that's when I shut it down. I know you're thinking, what a horrible tease. Yeah, so what? I am!

But actually I shut it down because I thought, do I really want this headache in my life? He has three kids and he's going through a divorce. I looked over at him and said, 'I'm sorry, this is not right for me. You have way too much baggage.'

He looked back at me with his big smile, showing off his gorgeous pearly-white teeth and said: 'You know what, Cap? I do have too much baggage and I understand why you don't want to get involved with me and I don't blame you. I don't think I'd want to get involved with someone in my position either.'

On that note, we hugged each other and we went our separate ways for the night.

Ty and I hung out together the next day. It felt like he was one of my best friends in high school. It was just easy to hang out with him and we loved each other's company. There was no mention of our conversation the night before.

Later that night Steve and Andrea asked us to go to a charity auction with them. They were to be guests of John Travolta and Kelly Preston and they asked us along. It was very exclusive and there weren't many people there. During the auction Ty asked me to bid on his behalf. He's very private – not like me, loud and proud. He's very reserved and I realised quite quickly that this is one of the things I loved about him. As I got to know him more and more he kept ticking all the boxes. The auction started and I made the bid on his behalf and later John Travolta and Kelly came over to us and said thank you for his generosity.

I think all this was very new to Ty. He was never really exposed to the entertainment world and he loved how alive and free and uncomplicated I was. We were having fun, pure and simple.

After dinner we went to grab a cup of tea because the thought of more alcohol made me want to vomit. We were both pretty wrecked from the night before. As we sat down in this cute little cafe in the Wynn hotel and had our green tea with honey, I asked Ty why he didn't call me right away after we'd met at Shoreditch House because I'd thought we'd got on really well that night. He told me, 'We did, Cap, but I was scared to get involved with someone with your level of profile'. He continued: 'It's quite intimidating watching the people coming up and asking for your autograph.' There had been quite a few paparazzi snapping away as we left Shoreditch House.

He's a very private person and being in the public eye just didn't appeal to him. He thought the only way any kind of relationship could happen between the two of us would be if we could meet up anywhere outside of England and he said he'd known that at some point our paths would cross again.

I thought, 'Wow, not only is he gorgeous but he's sensible too. I think I hit the jackpot here!' After he explained the whole thing we didn't discuss the future. I wasn't interested in it – I only cared about right then.

We continued talking for another hour but we were both hungover and tired from the night before so we called it in quite early. I gave him a huge hug and a gentle sweet smooch on the cheek, and we parted ways.

I woke up the next morning around 11am and experienced a feeling I've never felt before in my life. I missed Ty, but I missed him in an entirely different kind of way. I loved hanging out with him and when I was with him I didn't want to be with anyone else or be anywhere else. You know what it's like sometimes when you're on a date for a first time or when you've been with a guy for a while and you start daydreaming about someone else? It was not like that with Ty.

There wasn't anywhere else I wanted to be other than hanging out with Ty Comfort. It wasn't complicated, he wasn't calculating, it was unconditional and very real to me. Oh my god, was this the beginning of love? Not lust but real love. The everlasting kind? No. I just met him two seconds ago, it couldn't be, could it? That's ridiculous.

Ty called me the second he landed and we went out to dinner as soon as I got back to London, and all that bollocks about 'let's be best friends' went out the door because we ended up making out. And from that day forwards we were inseparable and the 24-year-olds could go take a hike.

In August Andrea and Steve invited us to go on holiday with them on their gorgeous mega-yacht, which was moored in St Tropez. We stayed with them for five days and then straight from the boat we flew to Ibiza, where we rented a six-bedroom house and invited a group of friends that included Ray, the guy who'd introduced Ty and me. It was a beautiful villa overlooking the sea in the best location and we had an amazing time. We laughed, we partied, we talked and made out non-stop. It was simple and we were having great fun.

We were there for ten days and on the last day we went for a final hurrah and it got messy. We had a party in a club and by the time we got back to the house I had to pack everything and Ty rushed me to the airport. When I got there I realised I'd got my timings completely wrong – I was still drunk, I couldn't string a sentence together and, yes, I missed my flight.

Ty took charge and booked me on another flight to southern Turkey, which was where I was heading next to stay with my best friends and their children. Ty, meanwhile, was going to Italy for a holiday with his children.

I finally arrived in Turkey 16 hours later, absolutely battered. Tired, hungover and missing Ty. I was staying with my friends Isis and Carlos. I'd known Isis for 16 years, since arriving in England. They'd sent me a driver to pick me up from the airport and take me to their yacht.

When I arrived, I was open-mouthed at the sight of the luxury before me. I was shown to my suite and the room was top-to-toe mahogany; the sheets on my bed were Pratesi – in other words they were £2,000 a set. All the bath products were from Bulgari – every detail was perfect. The chef came down shortly afterwards to get my dietary requirements. I told him I was vegetarian and he said, 'No worries, anything in particular you want for the morning?' I told him I loved Thai food and he said, 'I actually specialise in that'. Oh my god, here I am on this yacht in the middle of the ocean with this chef who specialises in Thai food, one of my faves. This is too cool.

And it was great to see Isis and Carlos, of course; we were all excited to see each other. I woke up the next morning to hear Calvin Harris blasting across the three levels of the boat, the seawater was so blue and the tender was out and ready for me to go for a ski. I needed that because my head was still throbbing from the day before.

I jumped into that crystal blue water, got on the monoski and my headache was soon a thing of the past. When I got back to the boat of course the interrogations started.

They wanted to know everything about this new chap in my life. They could tell I was glowing and that this relationship seemed different from the rest. Their insatiable appetite to hear all wasn't easily satisfied in one day.

But as the days went on, I didn't hear from Ty and I was worried. Blockbusters started up in my head. Maybe he doesn't like me, should I call him? No, I don't want to call him, I think men should be the hunters, not women. If he wants to talk to me he should call me ... But between you and me I probably dialled his number about 500 times without pressing the 'call' button.

We didn't talk the whole time I was away on the boat, and I thought for sure we were over. Maybe the 24-year-olds were bombarding him and he finally succumbed. After ten days, no texts, nothing. Towards the end I started moping around and Isis couldn't believe what she was seeing as this was a new Caprice. This was different. She knew I really liked Ty.

Everyone was quite concerned. I tried not to think about it because I didn't want to ruin anyone's holiday but who was I kidding, I missed him.

On the final day, still no word from Ty. We took a private plane, a Challenger, back from Turkey with all of our 30 (yes, 30!) bags on board.

I've been on a lot of private planes over the years so I know the ones I wouldn't be happy climbing aboard. I'd once taken a Challenger to the Bahamas, many years ago, for a party. It was just me on the plane and there was a massive thunderstorm. I promise I've never been so scared in all my life. The pilot told me, 'We could go back to Miami or I think I could land the plane.' I sat with my head on my knees and just prayed like crazy. We were swinging backwards and forwards and bumping around all over the place. It felt like lightening was hitting the plane and finally, after a turbulent landing, we arrived safely. Anyway, to cut a long story short, I know these planes are solid.

We arrived at Luton Airport's private hangar, unloaded the bags and were on our way back home when suddenly my phone rang. It was Ty. Everyone started screaming, including myself, but I told everyone to shhh and by the time I'd finished shushing everyone I'd missed the damn call. It was a disaster. What should I do: wait for him to call me again or call him back? So Isis finally interjected, 'Stop with all the "hunter"bullshit – just call him back.'

So I called him back from the car. It really felt like I was a teenager all over again – I was so nervous. He answered the phone right away and one of the first things he said was that he really missed me. Oh my god, relief. But then with the next words out of his mouth, my heart fell to the floor.

He said, 'I need to see you tonight, I need to talk to you.' Oh god, is this the end? He's going to give me the one liners I've given my ex-boyfriends in the past: I think you're a great guy but… this just isn't right for me, it's not about you it's about where I am in my life right now. Oh god, was this retribution?

I got home and unpacked, showered and put on my best frock; at least if I was going to get dumped I wanted to look hot… maybe he'd reconsider. The phone rang and my concierge told me Ty was there to pick me up. I told him to let Ty in and I could hear his footsteps approaching my door. My heart was pumping faster and faster and faster. Maybe

I needed to do a shot of vodka just to calm my nerves… I approached the door and opened it.

Oh my god, he looked so handsome. He was tanned and glowing – all 6ft 4in right at my door. I just wanted to tear off his clothes to be honest. Instead I very politely asked him to come in. I asked him if he wanted something to drink and he said no. I looked at him and couldn't think of what to say. I looked down at the sofa and that's when I thought, 'Oh god, it's coming now, here were go.' He looked up at me, his left hand reached out and gently grabbed my face and he pulled me in for a sensual kiss.

And then it got increasingly more intense. Well I'm sure you can figure out what happened next. Holy smoke, this was not what I expected.

Two weeks of continuous doubts, pining, worrying – all for nothing. I wanted to smack myself. I'd been with my closest friends on one of the most beautiful places on earth and I'd ruined it. I was just mad at myself. And I was also relieved.

At that point the words that came out of Ty's mouth next, stopped me in my tracks.

'I think we should move in together,' he said. So naturally, the dialogue running through my head went something like: should I play hard to get, should I decline?… No way. I said yes right away!

However, I had to be honest with him. 'I know we're only two months into the relationship but I have to be upfront about this: I want children and I don't want to get any deeper into this if that is not on the cards for you. Don't worry, I think you're an amazing human being and we could be best friends, I'm really cool like that, Ty.' I am such a damn liar.

I would have been gutted but I had to be direct about something as important as this.

Ty looked into my eyes and told me he'd suspected this would be the case and although he hadn't foreseen having more children he said: 'Let's go for it.'

Chapter 11

The Love Bug

I've mentioned my habit of meditating – I now do this every day of my life, even if it's just for five minutes. I'm so well practised that I can slip into it very easily and it makes everything calmer and clearer to me. One of the things I'd meditated on for a while was my 'perfect' man.

Nobody's perfect but I wanted someone who was going to understand me, whom I'd love being with and whom I could see a future developing. I had a sort of checklist of attributes – on a purely superficial level, he, of course, had to be hot. And tall! (By the way, I know it must be annoying I say hot about 1,000 times in this book!). Beyond that, of course he had to be intelligent, kind, ambitious… My list was very, very long. I felt certain that if I meditated for long enough, the right person would come into my life. I wasn't stressed about it, I knew it would happen at some point; I just had to be patient.

I had a feeling that Ty was that person. The right person. I'd never had feelings that strong for a guy – there were no doubts.

I knew that I wanted to be with him. It was of course, also down to timing. I'd been too wild and unsettled until then to contemplate anything really serious. But I was calmer now, more focussed, and the relationships I'd had before paled in comparison with this.

I was walking on air. I'd waited 39 years for this amazing man! We moved in together almost immediately and I think there were quite a few shockwaves amongst the Chelsea crowd who knew us! Up until very recently, Ty had been dating a number of gorgeous women and living in his bachelor pad. All of sudden he was in a serious relationship with me – serious enough for us to set up home together – and it caused a few ripples. I mean, I'd snapped up the hottest new bachelor to appear in this crowd for years!

Ty would be giving up his prized apartment. It was the envy of all bachelor pads, decorated by Philippe Starke with the walls covered in beautiful artwork. But it was very impersonal and there wasn't a single sign of femininity in that place – I'd open the fridge door to find nothing but vodka and cranberry juice and a cupboard full of vitamins!

We decided to rent a house in Notting Hill as I'd been living there for many years. We wanted to get a good idea of where we would live permanently before committing to buying a place. There was no suggestion we were just testing the idea of living together. From the moment we started to share our home together, it worked for us and we were so happy. By this time I'd met his children and we got on from the start. I wanted to make sure our permanent home had plenty of space for them to stay whenever they wanted.

In early October we decided to go to New York together for a few days because Ty had meetings out there. It was so romantic, I was on cloud nine with my new man: he was absolutely gorgeous in every way and I was so in love, over the moon I'd finally met my soul mate. We stayed in the Crosby Street hotel in a beautiful suite. We spent a couple of days walking around the city and Ty had invited his brother for a drink so he could meet me.

As Stuyvie walked into the lounge where we were sitting, I was shocked. He was about six feet, beautiful blue eyes and blonde hair, medium build. And what came out of my mouth, completely unbidden? 'Oh my goodness, Stuyvie, you aren't the geek Ty implied you were!' Ty looked at me in horror. I wanted to hit myself. The first time I met any of Ty's family! Even though it was true, why do I always have to be so obnoxious as to spit out the first thing that comes to my mind?

Thankfully Ty forgave me and Stuyvie laughed it off. We got on like a house on fire after that. We spent our time in New York meeting up with friends and just generally loving spending the time together. We fell more deeply in love every day. Everyone could see how happy we were, it was sort of infectious I think. A real case of: uh oh, here come the blissed-out couple again!

Later on that month, we threw a huge party for my fortieth birthday – it couldn't have been more different to my thirtieth, which I'd tried to ignore. This time it was a massive celebration with all my friends.

We took over the Cuckoo Club in London for the night and hired one of Pasha nightclub's (in Ibiza) resident DJs, who flew in from Amsterdam.

It was the Best. Party. Ever. It started off with a sit-down dinner and I had all my friends from the last 15 years of my life fly in for this big celebration. Everyone was in fancy dress because it was just before Halloween and it was just fantastic. Ty and I were very loved-up and you could sense the love and support around us. Everyone was so happy for us and our new budding relationship.

We had these hilarious guys called Faces of Disco who'd been in Britain's Got Talent that year and were utterly brilliant. We also hired a naked fire dancer and four bur-lesque dancers. Our DJ got everyone in a crazy party mood (although maybe the 40 magnum bottles of vodka helped as well). We didn't miss a beat at this major rager, it was a great way to bring in my forties.

On every table there was a big fat magnum bottle of cham-pagne and when that ran out it was replaced with another big fat magnum… it was a disaster (in a good way!), there was no chance you were getting out of there without being wasted. Poor Elen Rivas fell over, Sonique exposed her breast as she got into a cab… it was carnage, but what a great night!

A couple of weeks after my birthday I realised my period was late. I couldn't believe it. Surely I couldn't be pregnant that quickly? I did a pregnancy test and when that little blue line showed through I nearly did a dance in the bathroom. But I was in shock, too. Because although I'd been taking my vitamins and looking after myself really well on some level I couldn't believe that I could fall pregnant within weeks of trying.

That night, Ty came home and I said, 'I have something to tell you.' And he knew straight away what I was going to say. 'You're pregnant? That's fantastic!' We were just so happy! It was surreal, as it probably is for most women, I imagine. That dawning realisation that you have new life inside of you, that you're going to create a baby! It's amazing and daunting and wonderful and terrifying all at the same time.

No one knew anything about it. We were bursting to tell people but for now, we thought we should wait until that obligatory 12-week scan to make sure everything was OK. And why shouldn't it be OK? I had only just turned 40, I was fit and healthy and so was Ty. There was no reason to think anything would go wrong.

Meanwhile, all the early signs of pregnancy were kicking in with a vengeance. I felt nauseous and exhausted, my breasts were very tender – all signs that the pregnancy was progressing as it should do. I'd been taking folic acid, the so called 'building block' of new life for a few years as part of my recovery from Chronic Fatigue Syndrome, as well as about a million other vitamins and minerals. I'd looked after myself and I felt well, if tired.

Ty and I were in a special little bubble of our own private joy and I couldn't wait for the day we were able to share the news with our friends and family. All my dreams were coming true – the perfect man, the family and the life I'd always wanted.

We scheduled the appointment for the first scan and I got on with working, eating properly and getting a lot of sleep. I couldn't believe how exhausted I felt. This was not the Caprice of old – where was the wild child now? I trusted my body to get on with the job and started, tentatively, planning my future as a mother.

One morning, just before Ty left for his office, I got out of bed to go to the loo and found I had some spots of blood. I tried to stay calm but of course, my instinctive reaction was terror. I think it's natural to assume the worst, especially with a first pregnancy. I spoke to my friend Tara Sinnott – a really good friend of mine who was my agent for work in Ireland, although she's moved to LA now. She was so wonderful and really helped me out when I was going through tough times. Tara reassured me it wasn't unusual to 'spot' like this during a pregnancy but she did advise me to try and sort out an appointment to have an antenatal scan at the clinic.

I thought everything was going to be fine – I had no reason to think there would be any problems but I booked the appointment and Ty arranged to come with me. It was supposed to be this wonderful time when we would see our baby for the first time. The next day, we made our way to the clinic and the ultrasound department. The sonographer explained that the scan can take up to 45 minutes to make all the checks they need to make, and she asked me the date of my last period so she could establish how many weeks pregnant I was.

As the freezing cold gel was applied to my stomach, I tried hard to relax, but I was gripping Ty's hand for dear life. After about five minutes – which seemed like five hours – the doc said the chilling words: 'You should have a heartbeat by now.' She went on to explain that we might have our dates wrong, in which case the baby wouldn't be developed enough to detect a heartbeat.

I went back to work in a daze. Ty was convinced everything was fine but I was so upset, I didn't know what to
think. This is the minefield you enter when you start the
pregnancy process, the lurch from high to low as well as
the constant nagging worry I now had. This is what took me
by surprise because I've always been pretty level-headed. I
don't know if it's hormones or just that your body is in shock
during a first pregnancy, but either way, I wasn't used to
feeling this way.

Over the next few days I tried to relax but the spotting continued. Not only that, my pregnancy symptoms disappeared,
but I told myself this too was normal, I was just moving into
the next phase. And then one day I woke up in so much pain,
I swear to god I have never felt pain like it.

I was supposed to attend my friend June Sarpong's charity
lunch at a restaurant ironically called The Hospital. I felt terrible about letting them down as I had to cancel.

I'd started to bleed heavily and the pain was so intense I
thought I was going to pass out. I looked as white as a sheet.
I called one of the girls from my office and she came to pick
me up in the car, to take me to Chelsea and Westminster
Hospital. When I arrived, they ushered me into a room away
from everyone else and they were so incredibly kind. I think
they realised I would be recognised and of course, going
through something so traumatic, you really don't want the
whole world to know about it. At this point there was blood
everywhere and I was vomiting because the pain was so intense – the nurse explained that I was having a miscarriage
and that there were two foetuses, which was partly why the
pain was so severe.

Through the curtain of physical pain the word 'twins' filtered into my awareness and as I lay there in agony, my heart felt as though it were breaking.

Several hours in – I have no idea how long I'd been at the hospital at this point because I was in such a daze – I continued to bleed everywhere and the time in between contractions got shorter and shorter. Ty, showed up and was at my side. At that point I couldn't talk and I had no strength to move. I was exhausted both mentally and physically. Ty insisted I get a morphine shot and he asked for a D&C (short for Dilation and Curettage, which is when tissue from the womb is surgically removed).

Shortly thereafter the doctor came in and put a morphine shot into my left shoulder; ten minutes later the pain was gone. After almost two days of continuous contractions and vomiting I was now left with reality: I'd just lost the two embryos inside of me. I cannot possibly explain the feelings of loss and sadness. My heart was broken. I was then admitted into the hospital and waited for a D&C.

I would be under general anaesthetic as it's a procedure that takes no more than a few minutes and a surgeon was needed, and it meant I had to stay in the hospital overnight.

Early the next morning, having eaten nothing for more than 24 hours, I was allowed to leave.

I don't remember much about that journey home or much of the following days. For me, the way I deal with things is to try and concentrate on what comes next, on coming up with solutions. I try hard not to dwell on the negative stuff because it doesn't help, there's nothing to be done about the past but you can try and change the future.

Once we were home I do remember sitting with Ty a few days in, and saying, 'OK, honey, I don't want to slip into some massive depression. Maybe there was going to be something wrong with our babies and that's why this happened. I don't know. But we wouldn't want to bring babies that aren't right into the world.' It was the only way I could find to justify the miscarriage and try to make myself feel better.

Ty and I knew that we needed to think about the future and it wasn't long before we decided to start all over again.

I buried myself in work and there was a lot to do because By Caprice was going from strength to strength. The horrible times we'd gone through after the recession and the total rethink about how I was running the business were paying off. As well as lingerie, I'd moved into swimwear and bedding, which I was selling through Very.co.uk, and I had plans to develop a sleepwear range, too.

And so I had plenty to keep me busy but I had my dark moments. I remember talking to my mom. 'I feel like a failure and this is all my fault for leaving it too late to have kids.' Sometimes the pain was indescribable and yet I knew I had to keep going. I'm someone who really appreciates what I have because I've worked so damned hard for it, and it was not a comfortable place for me to be, feeling vulnerable and scared for my future. Maybe this time around I wouldn't be able to find solutions.

Going through a miscarriage is a physically and mentally draining experience and it takes a lot of strength to keep going afterwards; to pick yourself up and concentrate on your family and your relationship and nurturing what you have rather than thinking too much about what you don't have. And yet… and yet at times I'd feel so inadequate.

I'd say, 'Ty, you just don't understand how I'm feeling. How can you know what I'm going through?' He'd look at me with sadness in his eyes and say, 'I can, I feel the exact same way.' The temptation to withdraw completely, from everyone around me was very strong but mom would tell me: 'The longer you stay in that depressed bubble, the harder it is to get out of it. You have to pick yourself up and get on with it. I've been there, in the depths of depression and if you let yourself spiral it will take everything away from you.'

I couldn't lose my man over this, I had to grieve, but he and I were still in a relatively new relationship. I worried: will this tear us apart?

I felt I'd failed Ty in some way, too. He could have anyone he wanted and instead he was with a woman who can't give him children – this is the kind of conversation I would have in my head. Making blockbusters out of the situation, just as I had with the drunk driving but it was really hard not to. I couldn't let it ruin my relationship and damage my soul. I wanted a child and I wanted a relationship with Ty because I loved him so much. Men want to fix things and Ty is fairly unemotional; I'm aware that there are differences between the way we react and on top of all this, your hormones are throwing a party inside you. Nothing feels the same as it did before but I had my man and we had a plan. I just needed to move on and make the most of the future.

On the media front, at least the press were good to me again. I think they could see I had left those wild child days behind me. They printed nice stories about Ty and me and seemed to appreciate the fact that I made my own money by working hard at a business I owned. I was doing some TV work at this time but not very much, I was enjoying time with my man, we were just really getting to know each other and we were looking for a home to buy together. I guess I was grieving in my own way.

What I'd been through – well, it had gone straight to my core. It made me understand so much more that feeling of absolute yearning for a child, which somehow gets stronger when you think it may not happen. My imagined future always had children in it and suddenly I doubted my body.

Then in the spring of 2012, Ty came home one night and told me about a great doctor his friend had used in America, who'd helped his wife to get pregnant after years of trying. Having researched the subject to death by this time I knew that because Ty and I weren't exactly young whippersnappers, we might need to have our embryos checked out thoroughly before impregnation, to give the pregnancy its best chance.

The specialist we found had such a staggering success rate. In fact, since finding him he's developed his techniques even more. My doctor's success rate is not normal – his estimate is anywhere between 70 and 95 per cent success rate, depending on the age of the woman, using their own eggs. He's a wonderful man and I hope he'll be a friend to my family forever, he helped us so, so much. In fact in the last year I have put eight friends in touch with him, all of whom had difficulties with pregnancy and tried multiple avenues. All eight are either pregnant or have had a child thanks to my doctor!

One of the main reasons for writing this book is because I want to be very open about IVF and the struggles I had with trying to have my babies. There shouldn't be a taboo around this or around surrogacy. I've found that by talking about it to other women, they've really opened up to me and shared their heartache. Women who've told me they've had three, four, seven rounds of IVF – they've all unanimously expressed shame, heartache and sadness after their unsuccessful treatment. Not only does your body go through hell hormonally, emotionally it's a roller coaster.

These people who were scared to death to talk about it and who felt like failures are now really open about it.

You need a support system and to be able to talk it through when you're going through this process. It's harmful to keep it bottled up inside. I want to do all I can to get rid of the taboo around talking about IVF and infertility issues.

I have kept the clinic's name confidential because I've had a lot of problems with journalists calling my doctors before, trying to get hold of personal information about me and my family. They've called up pretending to be my cousin or my mother. And at times they have succeeded – one of the receptionists got fired in the end for believing them and giving out information. It was not nice for them, or me.

There are some differences in the techniques and drugs used between the US and the UK. UK specialists will tell you that the US use more 'egg stimulation', which can lead to a risk of multiple pregnancies, but there are more risks involved in this for the mother and for the embryos. At the moment, the average success rate for IVF for a woman aged between 40 and 42 in the UK is only 13.6%* but in the US is even lower: 11.8%+.

But the doctors we were using had a far higher success rate and so we booked the flights and took the plunge. We were off into the great unknown…

* Human Fertilisation & Embryology Authority, UK, most recent figures (2010).
+ Society for Assisted Reproductive Technology, most recent figures (2012).
Recorded by official MET office stats) between Aug 13 - Aug 14.

Chapter 12

The Big Leap

It was a beautiful, bright, sunny day when we arrived at the doctor's office. We were shown into the kind of room you just don't get here on the wonderful NHS, it was beautifully decorated and professional looking and yet homely at the same time. Like a four-star hotel.

It felt good. This was an optimistic, thrilling time for us and we were in it together.

The doc was kind and understanding and explained everything to us, and we spent a long time going over our different options but the most important thing was to begin tests to find out if there was any reason for me to have trouble conceiving – and carrying – another baby.

He explained what we already knew: as a woman gets into her late thirties, fertility drops dramatically. And the eggs a woman does produce are less likely to be healthy. It might also affect the health of the embryo (that is the woman's egg fertilised by the man's sperm) if the man is over 35; his sperm probably won't be as healthy either. It was hard to hear, even though I knew the drill. I'd read everything I could over the previous months, ever since I'd miscarried, and I wanted to know now what could be done in our circumstances.

All of the time I was thinking, 'I have the time and money to do this, I can come to the best place and get the best treatment; how is it fair for other women who don't have this kind of access?'

Ty and I had what seemed like hundreds of blood samples taken over the next couple of days. It was like being in some kind of vampire movie! Every time I turned around there was someone waiting to take my blood again and again, so in the end I became almost blasé about it. 'Oh yeah, here's another needle, suck me dry...' This has to be done in order to check hormone levels to make sure your body is at the right stage of its cycle before eggs can be collected.

One of the first things they tested for was my follicle count. This is the number of follicles you have in each ovary, and it dictates how much they might need to adjust your hormone levels.

The follicle stimulating hormone (FSH) levels are all-important – if they're ten or above, you're screwed, but I was a four – which was great (and very unusual for a woman of my age apparently). I felt relieved, at least something was in good working order.

I tried to stay focused: we would work out the best next steps for us as a family and we were doing whatever was in our power to have a baby. It was all I could concentrate on, that and the dawning realisation that this might take a little longer than we first thought. Taking the specialist's advice, it seemed that for us, *in vitro* fertilisation (IVF) was going to be the best treatment but first we had to identify what the problems were, why it was that I'd had the miscarriage in the first place.

After the third visit to the doc, he identified what he thought was a key issue for me: the lining of my uterus was unusually thin, which meant that any embryo would have a problem embedding itself. Without getting too technical, the lining of the uterus should be around 8mm thick in order to have a successful pregnancy and anything less than this can cause problems. If I was to start IVF treatment then I'd be given oestrogen shots, aiming to increase the thickness of this lining by around 1mm a day until it was the right environment for the embryo to be implanted. This would take anything from ten days to six weeks.

Ty and I had already discussed the fact that IVF was a good idea for us. The whole reason for spending a fortune by going to this doctor was that he had a reputation for making sure only the very healthiest embryos were implanted into my uterus, meaning less chance of miscarriage. Sure enough, the doctor explained that to have a successful pregnancy, those viable embryos would be placed inside me once they'd started to develop, which is four or five days after the eggs have been retrieved from my ovaries and fertilised.

This all sounds like such a technical process, and it is. But what you don't really expect is how emotional you're going to feel. Ty and I were confronted with the fact that in the next couple of weeks we were going to be making a baby and with this doctor's rate of success, there was every likelihood that it would work for us.

But there were hurdles to jump almost every day, with appointments at the clinic and daily hormone injections that I had to give myself. I didn't mind giving myself shots too much but it was a little tricky because it needed to be done at set times during the day. I remember pulling over in my car one day and having to do it there and then! It looks so suspicious, like I was some kind of desperate junkie! Very glad no one pulled over to check me out that day.

The daily jabs didn't bother me too much but there are some side effects. I felt a little nauseous some days and I'd get headaches too. I was staying with my mom and trying to do as much work as I could at home but again, I wondered how on earth women manage when they're trying to keep IVF private and at the same time they're going to and from an office and trying to fit the treatment in around their jobs. It's really tough and as the days went by, it became more stressful.

Before egg collection could happen, my follicles had to have reached the right size, but there was a chance that the ovaries could be dangerously over-stimulated, and the IVF treatment would be stopped before we'd even got started – so I was really nervous at each appointment.

After two weeks of injections, I had to have one final 'horse shot' the day before the egg collection, called an HCG, which helps with progesterone and oestrogen levels.

This was a big needle which had to be injected into the right upper corner of my butt! It could be done at home as long as it went straight into the muscle and exactly where the doctor directed it. If you were to inject the shot at the wrong time – even by ten minutes – your eggs would drop: game over, the whole process up to that point wasted. Ty said he wanted to do it, and I have a photo taken in my mom's kitchen of Ty giving me this huge injection! It wasn't pleasant but it did mean we were ready to go to the next stage.

Oh my god, that day will stay with me forever. Going into the hospital for the egg collection was incredibly nerve-racking and not particularly pleasant. I had to wear one of those really attractive hospital gowns and remove all my jewellery because they were going to administer a general anaesthetic. This isn't always done, it's often a local anaesthetic, but in the States they like to put you under. I hate anaesthetics, even if I have to deal with pain – the fewer drugs I'm on the better – but I succumbed this time.

'Caprice, we have to tell you that there are risks involved in egg retrieval,' the doctor explained just before I signed the consent form. 'It's very rare but occasionally the needle used to retrieve the eggs may damage your bowel or bladder.' I was already nervous and now I was being told risks that I didn't even want to know about.

The egg retrieval works by passing a long, thin needle into the ovary to retrieve the eggs and, thankfully, they managed 18. The doctor then rinses the eggs and they're placed in an incubator, before being fertilised later in the day with the sperm.

There was no way around it, though. I'd signed up for this, literally. 'It's a good job you're the best in the business then.' I smiled. And off to the land of nod I went...

I woke up feeling incredibly groggy and sore and my stomach was really distended. It was so uncomfortable.

'Am I supposed to have a stomach the size of a watermelon?' I asked. It was really disturbing. Apparently this isn't unusual, you just have to drink lots of water and eat properly and wait for it to go down. It took longer than I expected but finally, days later, I was back to normal.

I went home and I felt so ill and tired I went to bed and pretty much stayed there for the next two days. I was still making calls, working on my laptop and so on, but I felt really wiped out. I'd been warned it would be a tough time but nothing prepared me for the next stage: the waiting game.

For them to retrieve 18 eggs was pretty good and we had really high hopes. 'Maybe we'll be able to have twins!' I said excitedly on a call to Ty, who by now was back in the UK. Every day the clinicians would be testing for egg quality and to see if they were developing OK. It takes between three and five days for the embryos to start multiplying before the transfer can take place unless, of course, there were none healthy enough to be implanted.

None healthy enough to implant? Surely that couldn't happen to us, could it? But as the days went by, first one would die and then a couple of others wouldn't be viable or were damaged and then more would go until... after five days, there was just one, single viable embryo. Just one. And I now admitted to Ty and to the doctor that I'd hoped for maybe five or six. I was 40, yes, but I'd been pregnant quite recently and I was fit and healthy, wasn't I? Just one? It seemed incredibly unfair.

Mom and I were determined to be optimistic though. We'd named the baby; we'd planned his or her entire future out by the time I went back to the hospital.

On day five after the fertilisation we were back – this time for 'embryo transfer'. My body was ready now to accept a healthy embryo, I'd taken my medicine, I'd completed the process and we were so excited. It was a wonderful moment going into the hospital and knowing that on this day, my baby would start to grow inside me. The doctor was cautiously optimistic – of course they weren't allowed to guarantee anything but he had a great track record and, hey, we'd done all the right things, hadn't we?

This time there was no sedation. They use a small catheter, which goes into the uterus and this momentous event takes just ten minutes – incredible!

I felt fine after the procedure, just excited and nervous all at the same time. But then began the longest ten days of my life. It was a kind of low-level stress. I could almost see the darkness out of the corner of my eye, that deep cavernous depression on one side and on the other, a wonderful glowing joy, with me stuck somewhere in the middle. This weird middle ground was where I stayed, in bed most of the time (although still at my laptop, of course), resting as much as possible in order to give the embryo the very best chance to 'take'.

I'd convince myself I was pregnant because I thought my boobs hurt or I was craving lemon cake – yes, that definitely meant I was pregnant! And I felt light-headed so it had definitely worked, or I felt really tired, which meant my body was getting into its stride for the new baby. My mind literally ran through every single symptom of early pregnancy, justifying it, identifying it and wanting it so badly it hurt.

On the tenth day, I drove myself to the doctor's office. I kept thinking, 'Oh god, what if I'm not pregnant?' You could have cut the tension in the car with a knife. The doc had to take some blood to see if I was pregnant or not and then we had to wait a while for the results. He told me to drive home and he'd call when he received the results.

The phone rang when I was driving the car home. I had to pull over to take the call. I remember the traffic was really heavy, it was hard to stop the car and my stress levels were through the roof. I had to hear the doc's voice. 'I'm so sorry… you're not pregnant'. My heart plummeted and my tears fell, unchecked. I was so sad, so discouraged – I just needed a moment in silence to collect myself.

Chapter 13

If at First You Don't Succeed...

I had to call Ty and tell him the news. I just wanted to fly home as soon as I could, get back to him and lick our wounds together. My mom was terribly upset too, she'd been through the whole process with me and she'd seen how much I cared about this and how desperate I was to have this baby.

You know, though... somehow it wasn't as bad as going through my miscarriage. On balance, that was far worse and more devastating. I don't know why, maybe it was because the first time, I'd not been pregnant before and I didn't expect anything to go wrong. I also went through so much pain physically, it was very debilitating.

This second time, with the IVF, I'd been warned that it might not work and I'd researched it enough to know that my chances weren't brilliant. I got back to the UK and I sat with Ty, talking about and grieving for the life that wasn't meant to be. But for some reason, it didn't feel like the end. It felt as though we'd launched ourselves into some kind of fight and we weren't going to give up, not yet anyway.

'We have to try this again,' he said. I looked him straight in the eye and agreed. He knew how important this was to me and how I saw this child as part of the development of our family unit. Ty had his children but he was generous enough to know how much I needed to have my own child. I still felt such a failure – this was something I'd always wanted to do and because I'd waited too long, it wasn't going to happen for me. I was too old to have my partner's children. I knew he loved me and I loved him but I still felt this burden of guilt: I was putting him through all of this emotional roller coaster when he could have been shacked up by now with one of those ladies he was dating when he met me!

Within a couple of weeks I was back into my next cycle of IVF. The doc told me it's best to just carry straight on as with each month, the chances of conceiving reduce even further. This time I administered the shots myself whilst we were still in the UK. I was something of a veteran at it by now and after another week I flew to America to complete the treatment. This time, I was aware of everything: I had asked them not to give me the 'pre-med' to make me woozy before I went under, so I remember how cold the operating theatre was and I remember talking to the doc and laughing about what was going on: 'How many are you going to pluck out of me this time?' I asked him…'I'm guessing at least 18,' he said…and that was the last thing I remember.

I woke up in the recovery room and felt fine, but anxious. How many eggs this time? The doc arrived a few minutes later and said, 'OK, don't worry about anything but we have a few less this time: 15 of them, but there will be some strong, healthy ones there, I'm sure'. And so again, we had to wait for the next four or five days to see just how many would be healthy and strong enough for egg transfer into me. Every day it went down and down... along with my spirits. By day four I was convinced we wouldn't have any. Then what would we do? It could mean egg donation by a stranger, not something I was keen to do.

By day five, we had two viable embryos. Amazing! Two was good, two meant we had double the chance we'd had last time. But the doctor said, 'If I were you, I'd suggest you do one more round because your eggs aren't getting any healthier.'

This third round of IVF produced just one healthy embryo. Just one. My heart sank because no matter what we did, it seemed to make little difference. The reality is, the older you get, the harder it is to produce healthy eggs. We still had two others frozen, ready and waiting to be implanted along with this one. The final gamble – would it be worth it?

'I have never gotten anyone over the age of 45 pregnant using their own eggs.' My doc admitted this to me. I understood perfectly: we had to be very, very careful with the next step we took.

He sat me down and said, 'I need to talk to you about something that's concerning me. The lining of your uterus is quite thin, which makes it very difficult for the embryos to embed. It's because of this you're going to have a hard time getting pregnant.'

The doctor continued: 'There's good news and bad news. The good news is that you have healthy eggs, which is unusual for women in their forties. The bad news is that we could keep on putting healthy embryos in you but I don't know if they're going to embed themselves and if they don't it will result in another miscarriage. Your options are starting to decrease at quite an alarming rate and so, I just want to offer another option.

'What I'm suggesting is that we could use a gestational carrier to carry your baby for the nine months of the pregnancy. Or as people call this in the commercial world, a surrogate.'

The words hung in the air. It took a minute to grasp what he meant. The doctor had put this idea to us in a gentle but matter-of-fact way. A carrier – or gestational carrier – is the term used these days for a surrogate and the truth was, no, it had never occurred to me to use a carrier and I was taken aback – if not slightly horrified.

Up until now I had wanted to carry my own child, why the hell would I want someone else to do it for me? I had this niggling idea in the back of my mind that carriers were used by those women who just didn't want to gain weight and ruin their perfectly toned figures that took years to achieve and maintain. But I didn't care what pregnancy did to my body – I wanted to feel myself getting fatter as the months went by so I could feed my child. I would embrace the stretch marks and the milk-filled boobs if it meant I could carry a baby to term.

Suddenly, there was another option and this was going to take some time to get my head around, as it would do for Ty. The doctor suggested we go back to England to think it over and come back to him for more information if we needed it.

The journey home was a combination of sadness over the fact I wasn't returning pregnant, tinged with something else

– hope. Up until now it would have felt like a tragedy to me that I couldn't carry my baby but maybe it didn't have to be a tragedy at all. This was something I'd never considered but if it was the only way I could have a child then I definitely had to reconsider and thank goodness I had such a supportive partner who understood my yearning and was open to a very unconventional idea.

We did, of course, have a lot of concerns, the most important of all being: what if the carrier decides she wants to keep the baby after going through the pregnancy and birth? We worried about how it works trying to bring your baby home once he or she is born, when someone else has given birth to them. We worried about the story getting out and what people would say, so much to worry about and, at the time, it felt there were no guarantees of success. This was such a huge journey to embark on.

I couldn't understand why anyone would willingly go through surrogacy – after all, our bodies are supposed to be able to carry a child and to give birth, it's a natural process. Some people have thought I was doing it because I didn't want to wreck my body or because I couldn't take time out of my busy schedule. To me, that's just detachment parenting and I don't get it. But now, at this point in my life, with my dream tantalisingly close, I felt on the brink of something wonderful, even if it was pretty terrifying.

Ty and I needed to run this past our families before we made the final commitment because it was important they felt comfortable with it. It wouldn't have changed anything, we would still have gone ahead, but to have their acceptance meant a huge amount to us.

Thankfully, and quite surprisingly, my nervousness about telling people was misplaced. The whole family was really supportive. They all said, 'Go with the carrier, you have to take this chance.' They'd watched us suffering over the previous 18 months and they knew what we'd been through so far trying to have a baby, and as long as the legal side of it was all tied up, they had no problem with it. After all, as my carrier herself would say at the beginning of our relationship: 'What's wrong with having a babysitter for nine months?'

Everyone knew that our chances of being able to have a baby through IVF were getting slimmer and slimmer and that this was, in a way, our last shot and it was such a joy to us that they were totally on our side. My mom, who'd been with me every step of the way throughout the IVF and knew the agony I'd been through when I'd miscarried the twins, jumped at the idea! 'Do it. If that's what it takes and as long as you're happy with it, I'm happy with it.'

She offered to be the US 'link' if the carrier needed anything because, by this point, we'd decided we wanted to go with an American agency. One of the reasons was privacy: I'd tell the world what I was doing because, as in the cases of Nicole Kidman and Sarah Jessica Parker, short of faking it, people can see you've not been pregnant. But I'd tell everyone when I was ready – not when some little parasite decided they wanted to make a few quid and sell their rendition of my story to one of the newspapers.

I also liked the idea that the carrier would be able to just get on with her pregnancy in peace. Imagine if that story had broken here in the UK: the hunt would have been on for my carrier immediately. I wasn't prepared to put anyone through that.

With a reputable surrogacy agency, every potential carrier is screened beforehand and agencies will not have a woman on their books who hasn't been screened for a variety of conditions including HIV and hepatitis. Not only that, they will also have a set of requirements that might include things like a history of drug use, a difficult pregnancy or smoking. My agency also specified the carrier should have had a successful pregnancy before and now actually be raising that child (or children).

It was all becoming so real...'Are you ready for this?' I said to Ty, smiling nervously at him as we received our potential carrier's details.

'I don't know, ask me nine months down the line!' he grinned.

We had a pile of potential ladies' résumés to go through. As we began looking into surrogacy, we came across some truly terrible stories coming out of India, Thailand and Malaysia, where women are basically paid peanuts to carry a child for a western couple who aren't able to have their own children.

These places are almost like baby 'farms' with stories of women being implanted with multiple embryos in order to ensure a pregnancy and then having to terminate one or more if the implant results in a multiple pregnancy. I've also heard stories of babies being mixed up at the hospitals, fee discrepancies (ie parents being totally ripped off with no comeback) and the women themselves forced to live in very basic accommodation under some kind of surrogacy 'regime'.

This kind of experience was about as far away from my story as can be and because the infrastructure has been up and running in the States for a good ten years now, it takes the guesswork and the risk out of it. Of course, you always have this little knot of fear inside that something could go wrong, but the way we viewed it was that any pregnancy has risks of one sort or another and we were minimising the risks by finding the right woman with the right agency to do this for us.

The surrogacy agency came very highly recommended to me by my doctor in the States who said they were excellent, professional and sensitive. If you're going into a scary process like this, that's exactly what you need to hear, but Ty and I weren't just going to go on the say-so of one doc and we called a number of agencies to 'grill' them.

Where do you even start with something like this? You start with the basics and beyond that, you get a 'feel' for the kind of people you're dealing with.

My burning questions
- What's the exact nature of the process involved and how do you support the carrier and the parents throughout this process?
- How long has your company been in business?
- How many successful (ie without any problems at any stage) surrogacies have you achieved?
- Do you have any outstanding law suits that have resulted from surrogacy cases in your care?
- What are the psychological and medical scanning processes for your carriers?
- How much will this cost and how transparent are those costs – any surprises along the way?
- What about insurance – for the couple employing the carrier and for the carrier, how does all that work?

- How will you make sure we can be named as sole parents to our child?
- Is there a case worker who helps us throughout every step of the process?
- Does the agency personally visit and monitor our carrier throughout the whole nine months? Would the carrier be open to eating nothing but organic food, of course at our expense?
- Would the carrier mind one of my family members joining her at all the doctor's appointments?
- Would the carrier mind doing Skype throughout all the doctor's appointments at the doctor's offices?

The legal implications were of real concern to Ty and myself, of course. We live in Britain but both have American passports – it could get complicated. We didn't have anyone else to talk to about this either, so it was down to research, research, research. And a little bit of blind faith that everything would work out OK in the end, of course.

After making calls to several agencies, we did in fact work with the one first recommended by our doctor. I liked them because they were very sensitive to our needs – they knew it was a first for us and that it was a very big deal in our lives, and they understood that whereas some of the other agencies were far too much about the business.

They also seemed to care about the carriers on their books and knew a lot about each of their cases. They offered fantastic care throughout the woman's pregnancy, psychological help, regular support meetings and availability 24/7 if there were any problems. In short: they were people we trusted.

Surrogacy works in different ways depending on what the health issues of the parents might be. We would be using a gestational surrogate – which means she would be implanted via a process called intrauterine insemination (IUI) using the embryo created by my egg and Ty's sperm. In other cases a carrier might be implanted with an embryo created from a donated egg from a woman who isn't the biological mother, or an embryo created using both donor eggs and donor sperm.

There is also what's known as partial surrogacy, which is where the sperm from the father is used but combined with the egg from the carrier – the fertilisation process for this is done by artificial insemination or intrauterine insemination. We would never go down this road; that was just not an option for us. We still had my healthy eggs and a couple of years in hand for egg extraction from me.

And so, after filling in all kinds of details about ourselves and having long, investigative phone conversations with the agency – 'Are there any medical issues? What kind of parents do you think you would be? What did you have for breakfast? (Not really, but you know, it was very, very in-depth, as it should be) – we eventually signed a contract (which was, naturally, incredibly detailed) and we were sent a number of potential carriers to choose from. It was quite surreal, going through all these questions with the agency and having a pile of résumés to look at. On some levels it didn't feel real. Could we really become parents this way, by answering a bunch of questions and selecting someone to carry our baby?

Each carrier had filled in all kinds of medical details, lifestyle details and information about their general beliefs and outlook on life, so we could get a great picture of the kind of person we would be dealing with. It's a sort of dating agency experience but with more people involved. Utterly strange and yet there's something that makes you feel quite in control of the situation because you wind up knowing so much about the potential carriers.

You also see a photo of them and it's amazing how quickly you can form an opinion of someone when you have all this to go from. But it's so weird – you're sitting at home on the sofa mulling over who is going to carry your child and this person is a stranger, at least to begin with.

Some parents aren't interested in forming a relationship with their carrier but for me, it was absolutely vital I knew this lady and felt a part of her life for a while, and she needed to feel OK with it otherwise it wouldn't work. She was going to carry my baby – of course I wanted to know she was a good person and I needed to know how she was feeling throughout the pregnancy.

It was hard because there was a distance of 5,000 miles between us most of the time and yet somehow we managed it. And for us, it worked brilliantly.

We spoke to a few different women during this selection process but with one of them in particular we just clicked straight away.

So let me introduce you to the wonderful 'Tina'. Now, 'Tina' is not her real name because we have all signed a lot of confidentiality forms to protect her and to protect my children, but we'll call her Tina for the purposes of this book. To refer to her constantly as 'my surrogate' or 'my gestational carrier' sounds wrong, doesn't it? For someone who has played such a major role in our lives, I'd like her to have a name – even if it's not her real name!

We discovered Tina on the first day of trawling through the potential carriers. She was 32 and was (is) married with four (yes, four!) children of her own, all under eight. It seemed to me that Tina had all the best attributes and sounded like a lovely person. She had never been a gestational carrier before and this was the one thing that did worry us a little bit – it's usually better to have someone who has already been through the process, just as reassurance. But apart from this, she sounded wonderful.

Right up until the birth, all communication with a carrier is often done by email or phone, which is the way we did things with Tina. We had specified that we didn't want some-one who drank alcohol, we wanted someone who was fit and healthy and had really good moral values. Furthermore we wanted someone who had children already so that we knew she could carry a child to term. And someone who was will-ing to eat organic food only. Tina ticked all those boxes, and she came across to us as a warm, intelligent, down-to-earth lady who had all the right attributes but, importantly, we liked her. Ty, who's very instinctive, took to her straight away – she told us about her life as a full-time mom and why she wanted to be a carrier.

She said she'd discovered the one thing she had a real tal-ent for was having babies and because she's someone who gets a real sense of joy out of doing things for other people, to her, this was the ultimate way to do that. As she said, 'I wanted to help a family to experience the joy I've felt having my own children.' which was such a wonderful thing to hear.

She and her husband (who was fully on-board with the surrogacy) had already decided they didn't want to have any more children but as she was still only 32, she was going to use her child-bearing as a force for good. I thought she was an inspirational person to talk to – how many women can say they're doing this for those reasons? Ty and I completely believed her and we've been proved right because Tina is a very, very special lady. She kindly agreed to be interviewed for this book and I'm very grateful, it's good to be able to dispel some of the myths around surrogacy and for her to share her side of the story. I'd like to say I didn't edit any of her words. It was her experience and regardless if it was good, bad or indifferent I feel as you as a reader must not be misled. And here's the absolute truth in her words.

TINA'S STORY

'I always say that God gives everyone gifts and you're supposed to use those gifts to help others, and I joke that because I'm super-good at pregnancies and deliveries, that's my gift from God and I should use it.

I was 32 when I decided I wanted to try surrogacy: I have four kids of my own and I love being a mom but I have no desire to have any more children of my own and I really wanted to help another couple have their own family.

My husband was happy with the idea and he wasn't even particularly surprised. He knows what I'm like! I'm always volunteering for things, donating to charity and trying to help out as much as I can and this was a more extreme version of that. I knew very little about surrogacy at first but I did know a girl from my high school who worked at a fertility clinic and so I contacted her for some advice. I'm a Christian and my personal view is that I don't believe in termination of a pregnancy and I realised that this might be an issue for some surrogacy agencies but for me it was a deal breaker.

My friend told me there would be agencies who would refuse to take me on because of this but she gave me the name of the agency Caprice and Ty used, and this agency were happy to sign me up but warned me it could take a while to find parents who matched up with me and my specifications. I thought, that's fine, I'll give it a year and see what happens. If no one comes through then it's just not meant to be. In actual fact, it all happened very quickly.

First of all though, I had to go through the registration process, which is very thorough. It's not an application form as such, it's all the details about you, your lifestyle and your attitudes, so that the couple can feel really comfortable about the person who's going to be carrying their baby. I also had to write an open letter to potential parents explaining my motives for wanting to be a surrogate.

The agency explained that there would be shots (injections) and pills to take, in order to tell your body you're pregnant and kick-start that process. This was almost the end of the road for me before we'd even started – I hate needles! I'm deathly afraid of them. But then I thought, 'If someone told me that the only way I could get pregnant, naturally, was to have progesterone

*injections every day for eleven weeks, would I do it?' Yes.
I would do it without even thinking about it and so if I
needed to do it to help out a couple who couldn't have
their own child, that's what I would do. And that was it,
I tried to put aside my fear!*

*Caprice and Ty were the first couple I'd spoken to
and so I didn't really know what to expect from it. The
agency set up what's called a 'matching call' which is
exactly as it sounds: you get to chat with the parents so
that you can see how you get along. I thought they were
absolutely lovely people and we seemed to click very
quickly with each other.*

*The funny thing was, the agency told me we would
need to be extra discreet because Caprice had a high
profile. At this stage I only knew her first name and
I didn't know who she was but then it clicked – my
husband and I had watched a reality show years ago
called* The Surreal Life *and Caprice had been on it! We
remembered at the time that she had been very sweet on
the show. I thought she'd been the nicest person on there.
I wouldn't have said yes to somebody if I didn't like
them, no matter how much money was being paid.*

*I think Caprice and Ty liked me because I had a faith
– I doubt it would have mattered which faith it was –
it's just that it signified the fact that I had quite strong
morals and was unlikely to be a big drinker. Caprice
asked me of course how I would feel about handing the
baby over after the birth and I tried to reassure her as
much as possible that I was doing this for them, not for
me. In California, the law sides with the parents rather*

*than the surrogate, which means it's actually illegal to
hold onto a baby once you've given birth, but even so, it's
still a worry any parent will have.*

*You have to have a close relationship with the
biological parents for the trust to be there and because
you're making important decisions together with them. I
have heard of stories via other surrogates who've begun
the relationship well and then had problems further
down the line. One lady in particular said the mother
became very controlling the further into the pregnancy
the surrogate got. She even told the surrogate she didn't
want her to use a microwave!*

*In the case of Caprice and Ty, they couldn't do
enough for me, and were wonderful right from the
beginning. I was introduced early to Cap's mum as
she lives in California and would be around if I had
any problems. She's a wonderful lady and she told me
afterwards that she had liked my résumé the most out
of all the other potential surrogates, which was great. I
felt almost a part of the family – and it's a relationship
which has continued in the same vein.*

*Caprice and I had constant Skype calls, texts and
emails between us. It was tricky because of the time
difference sometimes but we kept in constant touch. I
had Cap's mom's phone number if I needed anything and
she came to the important clinic appointments with me.
I'd known from the outset that Caprice wouldn't be in the
country and I had to decide whether or not I was happy
with that but for me, as long as we had a relationship, it
made little difference – the outcome would be the same.*

I told my kids what was going on, as soon as I knew I'd been selected. I explained to them that there was a mommy who couldn't have a baby of her own because her tummy didn't work for growing a baby and that the doctor was going to put her baby in me and I was going to help it grow. I said that we'd then give the baby back to the mommy when it was ready. They'd just had some chicks hatch in their classroom at school and I asked them, 'Was the chicken the mommy who made the eggs or was it the incubator that helped keep it warm and grow the eggs?' and they said, 'The chicken.' They loved it – they were so excited and proud to tell people their mommy was a surrogate. I wanted to be a good example to my kids, that when you can do something and someone else can't, then you should help them if you can.

My extended family loved it and I didn't have any negative responses. Some people would say, 'I bet you got a lot of money for doing that,' and I'd hate to hear that. For the pain and suffering you go through, it's not a lot of money and after all, it's a service like performing an operation for someone. If a doctor can do surgery on your heart, do you begrudge him the money for what he's doing?

The medical side of the procedure went very well. Caprice had found a doctor who was very keen to use a more natural approach, which meant that rather than giving me pills to make the lining of my uterus thicker, he waited until my own cycle had reached that phase – his belief is the less medical involvement, the better. So I needed to be checked frequently to work out where

I was in my cycle and then, when I was ready, the fertilised embryos would be put inside my uterus. From then on, I had to be given meds so that my body thought I was pregnant. Luckily my wonderful husband gave them to me because I think I would have found it really really hard to do myself. These shots help your body to hold on to the growing embryo until your body takes over the pregnancy.

I felt fine throughout this time; all had gone well and although I was a little tired, Caprice had done something so wonderful for me. In the early weeks just after I'd had the procedure to put in the embryos, Cap called me and said: 'Mom and I have been talking and we've realised you're a stay-at-home mom with four young children and you're probably not feeling too great right now.' At first my heart sank, were they worried I wasn't capable of carrying their baby? In fact they said, 'We want to hire some help for you to make sure this isn't physically too much for you.' It was great! They actually hired someone to help out with the housework and so I could relax with the children and not stress about all the other things. She even offered to employ a live-in housekeeper but I really didn't want to take advantage at all and I turned that down. The other thing Caprice had specified in our first chats was that she wanted me to eat organic food because it would be so good for the baby. I was delighted – who wouldn't want to eat organic food if they could afford it? It's so expensive over here in the States. And this is where Caprice has really done something for my family.

*As the weeks went by I carried on buying my kids
'regular' food while I was eating organic and the thing
was, I would notice a huge difference in how quickly
my food would go bad compared to my kids' food. I
started to ask myself, what on earth is in this food to
keep it fresh for longer? What are they spraying it with?
It totally opened my eyes to the food industry and now
everything in my house is organic and it's changed
our lives. I really felt like she was doing the best thing
possible for her baby and it made me realise I wanted
to do the same for my family. It's kind of cool that I was
able to change her life and she was able to change mine.*

*The pregnancy was going along fine until we reached
my ten week scan. We knew by this time that there
were two babies in there, both embryos had 'taken'
and we knew there was a little boy and a little girl and
everything was fine. I knew one of the embryos was a
little smaller than the other and had a slightly slower
heartbeat but I didn't think it was a problem. Which
was why, when the doc broke the news to me that the
baby girl didn't have a heartbeat, I was so devastated.
I had no idea this was a possibility and I've never had
a miscarriage, and so to have four flawless pregnancies
and then this was a big shock. I was so upset for Caprice
and Ty because it meant they'd lost another baby; I
knew how upset they would be. It was a very, very hard
conversation and of course I had no idea at that time
Caprice was pregnant and that same day was bleeding
a little bit. I really can't imagine the pain she must have
been in on that day.*

But after that, everything else went really well. With your own pregnancy you're busy planning names, where the baby will sleep and getting everything ready but there were none of those things to consider for me and so I was able to enjoy the whole pregnancy experience without the extra stress. It was very different from carrying my own child: the kids would talk to the baby in my stomach and I remember going to the beach and them saying, 'This is the baby's first time at the beach!' They were so excited for Caprice and Ty but they knew all along that I was basically a pre-natal nanny.

I did fall quite ill at one point when I was about five months pregnant. The whole family had been ill with flu but I thought I'd got away with it. I was the last person to get it and because I was pregnant and maybe my immune system was compromised, I felt terrible. I had a temperature and I couldn't pee at all, I was so dehydrated. I know this is really dangerous when you're pregnant as it can bring on contractions and early labour so I went straight to hospital and they put me on an IV drip to make sure I got plenty of fluids. I was sent home quite quickly but then I woke the next morning with my heart racing and it wouldn't stop. It was very scary and my husband took me back to the hospital. Eventually they worked out that the flu virus had gone to my heart and this was making it race. I was kept in the hospital for a few more days and I begged them not to do any more tests than they needed to. All the while I was very conscious of keeping this baby healthy and I didn't want them taking any risks, as long as I was going to be OK, obviously.

It wasn't long after this that Caprice told me she was pregnant. I had actually guessed, having seen some pictures on the UK news websites of Cap in a bikini on a beach. But when she told me I was still pretty shocked; all I could think to say was, 'That's wonderful, congratulations!' That's genuinely how I felt, I was thrilled for her. And then my next question, before I could stop myself was, 'You do want to keep this baby too, right?' She replied, unsurprisingly: 'Of course we do, absolutely!' and she was laughing her head off when I said that. She'd been so worried about telling me, in case I worried about the future for the baby I was carrying. Caprice thanked me, in fact, for helping her to get pregnant! She said: 'Because I knew you were having my baby, I was finally able to relax and I'm sure I wouldn't have gotten pregnant if it hadn't been for you taking care of everything.'

It was such a wonderful surprise for everyone and I completely understood why she'd waited a while to tell me she was pregnant. She'd had a horrible time miscarrying and then having failed IVF so of course she was going to wait until everything was fine before telling anyone about it. She knew the story was about to come out in the media about my pregnancy and I soon became the 'American mystery woman' the papers were talking about in England. It was so funny, I remember saying to my husband, 'Who would ever have thought I'd be described as a mystery woman to anyone?'

Right at the beginning of my pregnancy, when I'd felt nauseous or very tired, I'd kept it from Caprice because I felt she might be sensitive to the fact that I was pregnant and she wasn't but from this point onwards, we talked constantly to each other about our pregnancies and it was so wonderful to be able to do that. She would ask me for advice and say 'I can feel this and such and such a thing is happening, is this normal?' and I'd be able to reassure her. It was a really wonderful time for us.

I warned Caprice that I have given birth to all my children at 38 weeks – full term is usually considered anything from 38-42 weeks but I seem to be on the early side. With this in mind she and Ty had decided to come over a month before the due date just in case, as she was so worried about missing the birth.

Maybe because I've had four kids, I start to dilate early, usually a few weeks before going into labour. I felt I ought to tell Cap it had started to happen, even though I knew labour would be weeks off. It did throw her into a little bit of a panic and within a few days she'd somehow managed to finish all her work and fly over.

My doctor at the local hospital was fantastic. She's delivered all four of my kids and she loved that I was a surrogate. She gave me medical clearance before I started the process and she was very excited for me. She really understood that Caprice and Ty were the parents and she was happy to talk to them over the phone during the pregnancy. Sometimes you get a situation where the docs are quite rude to the parents and will only speak to the surrogate but fortunately my doctor completely included Caprice and Ty because she knew they were just as important.

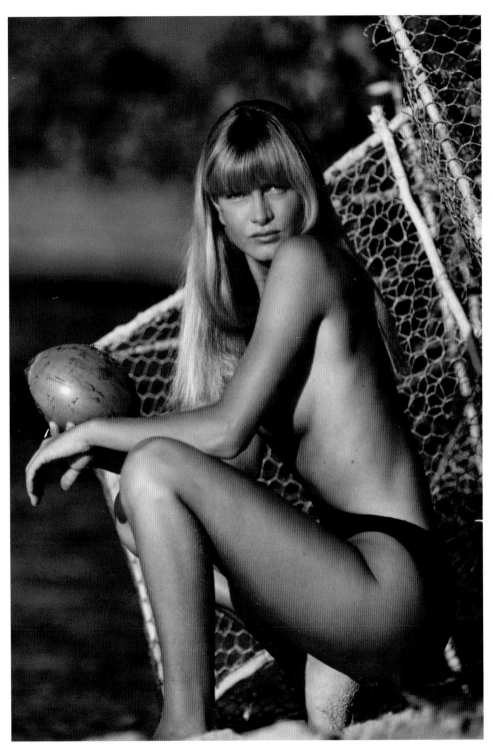

Above: My first modelling assignment when I was 19.

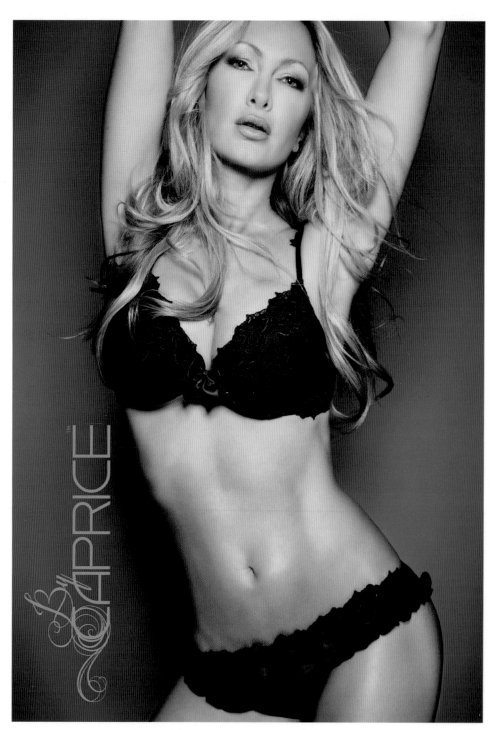

Above: Official 'By Caprice' campaign imagery.

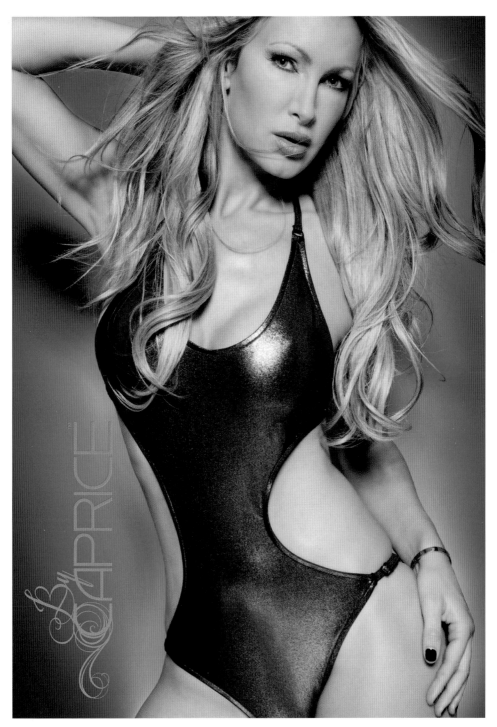

Above: Official 'By Caprice' campaign imagery.

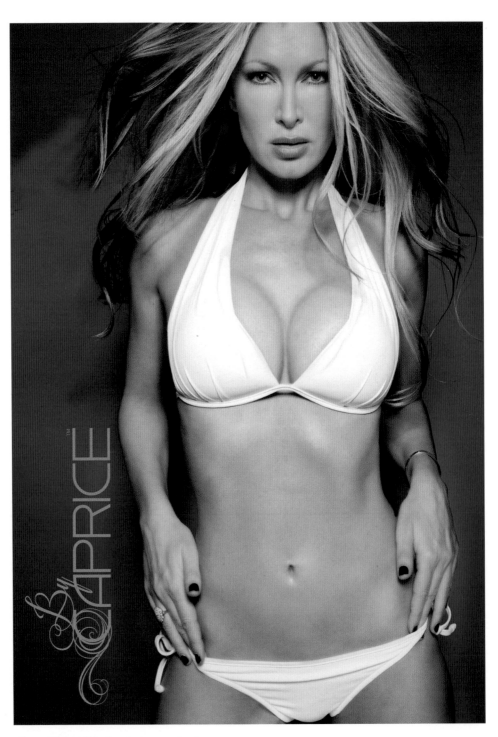

Above: Official 'By Caprice' campaign imagery.

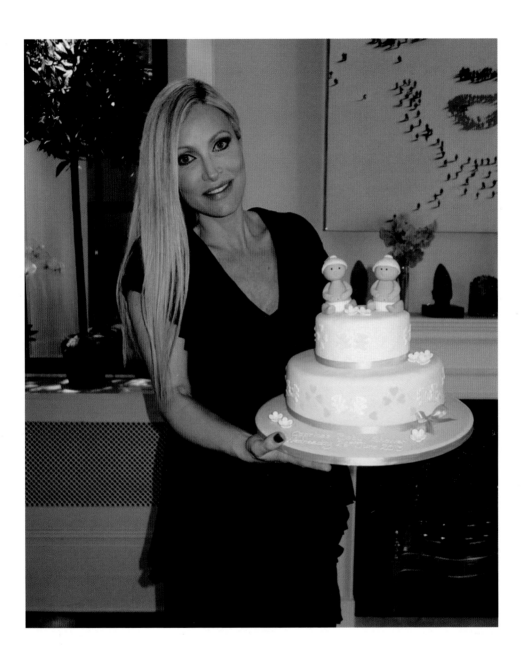

Above: My baby shower in 2013.

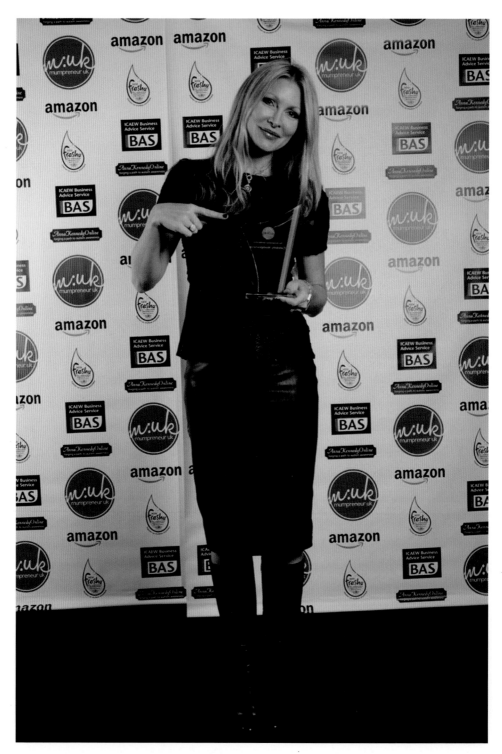

Above: I won Mumpreneur of the Year in 2014.

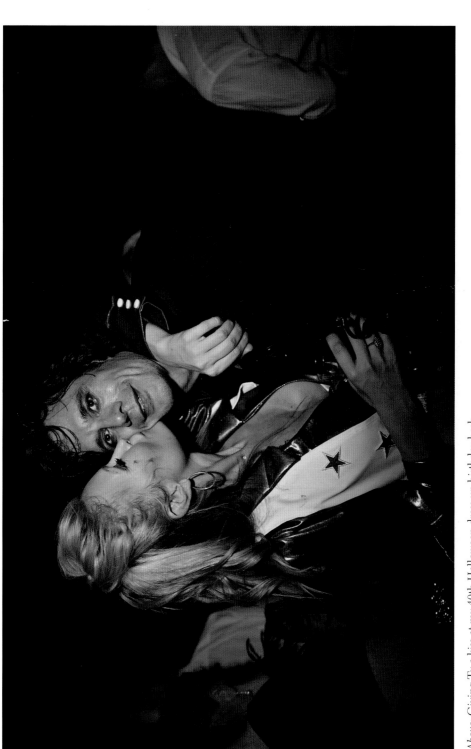

Above: Giving Ty a kiss at my 40th Halloween dress up birthday bash.

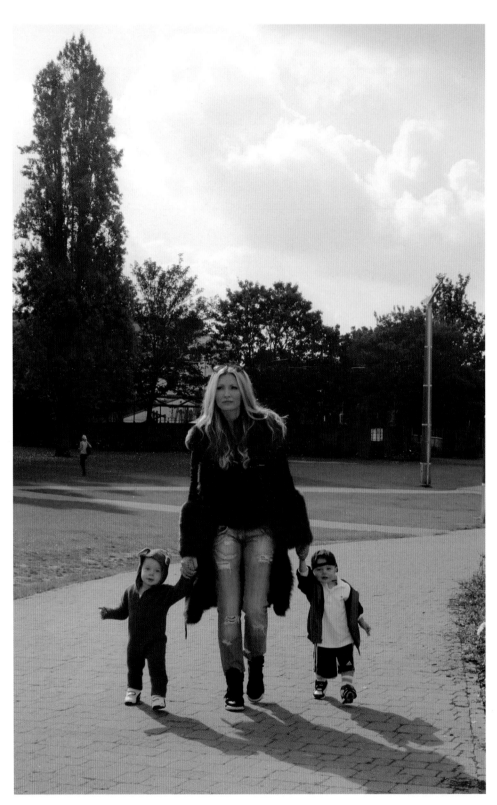

Above: My gorgeous boys.

The labour was all very straightforward – except that right at the last minute my husband disappeared to get something to eat and they had to call him over the tannoy. He appeared moments later clutching a quesadilla in his hand, it was so funny!

Caprice and Ty had a room at the hospital next to our room and her mom was there too. It was very sweet because I was all too aware that Caprice was due to have a baby in the next few weeks and so I was worried about her thinking there was anything wrong. As you're about to push, your body starts shaking and I held her hand and told her it was normal and she didn't need to worry.

It took only two pushes for the baby to be born and Cap was sobbing so much, she was just so happy. At that moment I felt such incredible joy. I remember saying, 'I wish I had a picture of this, this is the face I want to remember, the reason I've done this.' And then I realised, 'I'm done! I can take pictures!' So a few seconds after giving birth I was there taking photos with my phone! I was laughing as I did it, the room was so full of joy – I've never seen anyone so happy.

I knew how much I cherished the first moments with my babies and I wouldn't want anyone else touching them until my husband and I were ready. I wanted Caprice to have that experience and so I didn't touch the baby until they had. And it was a wonderful hour just sitting there watching her singing and talking to him, she was completely in her own world.

Of course I was worried I'd feel some sadness afterwards but I hoped the joy would overpower the sadness. But unexpectedly I felt no sadness, nothing at all. I told Cap it was as though I were her friend and I'd been lucky enough to be in the room with her when she gave birth. I was surprised at how I felt, even when I left the hospital the next day. I thought I'd feel sorrowful not to be taking a baby home but it was as if I'd been in hospital for some other reason.

I was able to go back to normal life very quickly and I rested up for a while. Caprice offered to extend my housekeeping by another six weeks after the delivery and so I was able to just rest and focus on my family while I recovered. She was so good to me, too good! I always say to her 'You've set the bar too high, no one will ever be as generous as you've been!'

My kids met the baby the day after he was born and then a couple of weeks on we met Caprice's second born son at the house. Caprice said right from the start that I'm their Aunty Tina and my husband is their Uncle and she said she wanted them to know us and we're part of the family now. When I see the boys now, I love them both the same and it's just like seeing my friends' little boys.

I have a picture of Caprice and me side by side just before we both gave birth and then another of us with the boys after they were born taken just a few weeks apart and each time we see each other we take another picture like that. I completely agree with her decision not to reveal which baby was from me and which was from her because people will make all sorts of judgements and jump to conclusions, which actually don't make any sense. She loves them equally so why differentiate?

Being a surrogate was the best experience ever. I loved it so much I'm actually pregnant with a baby I'm having for another family! When someone asks me how I can do this, they always say, 'Oh gosh, I couldn't do that, how can you give the baby up?' But my answer is: 'I'm not giving him up, I'm giving him back to his mother. I love being a mom, I couldn't imagine not being a mom and I want to help someone who couldn't do it.' How could you argue with that?

Chapter 14

The Curveball

I'm not afraid of much but I am afraid of heights. Just thought I'd like to make that clear before I explain how terrifying the idea of diving off a ten-metre high board into a swimming pool is to me.

And yet… and yet… something made me say 'yes' to a TV show called *Splash!* Probably my new manager, Vickie White.

Vickie (aka 'Vix') and I had worked together many years before when she'd been a TV producer. I'd not seen her for years but one night in mid 2012 I was at an awards show after-party when I saw this vision tottering towards me on her six inch heels, with cleavage jiggling and clutching a bottle of champagne. She was the epitome of Ab Fab's Patsy.

'I know that face…' I thought. 'Vickie, is that you?'

She screamed, 'CAAAAAAAPPPP!' She was wasted! She came straight over with the bottle of Bolly she'd apparently pilfered from the hotel's kitchens.

We caught up with each other whilst downing the fizz and that's when she told me she'd left TV production and set up as a talent manager/agent. Something clicked for me at that moment. I'd spent the last four or five years throwing everything I had into By Caprice but I had done very little in the world of entertainment; maybe it was time to get my name out there again – with the right project, naturally.

Olympic fever was at its height when ITV came to us with this new show, *Splash!* It was to be prime time ITV1 Saturday night. Vickie said to me: 'Cap, this show is going to be great – everyone will be watching it, it'll be a fantastic challenge for you and, hey, you get to show off all that gorgeous By Caprice swimwear into the bargain!' I was already a strong swimmer but I was really nervous about this project. What if I looked like an idiot on prime time TV? What if I fell off the diving board?

But then I heard Tom Daley was training the contestants and he was a real hero of mine and so I took a deep breath and signed on the dotted line. I didn't think too much about it at that point: it would be great to learn a new skill and, anyway, how hard could it be, learning to dive properly into an Olympic-sized pool? And I trusted Vickie's vision.

We were to have just eight days of full-time training spread over a two-week period with Olympic medal winner and all-round lovely guy Tom Daley at the Luton Sports Village. There were 13 celebrities in all including Donna Air, Linda Barker, Joey Essex and the boxer Anthony Ogogo. One of the contestants, Jennifer Metcalfe, dropped out at the last minute, which, if I'd only known at the time, was probably a wise move! I had no idea how tough that training was going to be; no idea at all. I remember walking in on the first day and seeing the lowest diving board, which was three metres and then looking up at the top board – ten metres. And Tom telling me that by the end of the training I'd be jumping off that one. I laughed – he had to be joking, right?

Tom shook his head with that big, smug grin on his face. We were all training all day, again and again climbing that ladder, practising our technique, jumping over and over again until we were black and blue all over. I was so beat-up by the end of it, I'm amazed you can't see the bruises on those YouTube clips of me diving. It took six days to train to do a one-and-a-half off the spring-board. This is one of the hardest technical dives to master. I asked Tom how long it would take if you were training to be a competitive swim-mer. 'Oh, about a year,' he said, the grin never faltering.

Holy smoke! And we were supposed to perfect this dive in ten days? This sounded totally insane. How the hell could this crazy production get insured for this?

We were staying at a hotel nearby. On the first night after the training I arrived exhausted, ready to crawl into bed at midnight.

As soon as I saw the place, the hairs on the back of my neck stood on end. The building dates back hundreds of years and it's huge and very imposing but as I walked through the doors I just knew there was a presence there – and not of the flesh-and-blood variety either.

I went to check in and I said, 'Look, is this place haunt-ed?' The receptionists looked uncertainly at each other and then back to me. 'Er, well, Miss Bourret, it has been known to have a few incidents'. Incidents? It had more than that.

That night it ran the gamut of haunting jiggery-pokery. I had no choice but to stay in my room because it was too late to check in anywhere else and besides that, it was just before Christmas so everywhere was full and I was seriously knackered from the training. I was shown to my room, which, by the way, was absolutely beautiful. Magnificent.

I decided I'd keep the TV on to keep me company and stop me feeling so, well, haunted. I was deliriously tired and I knew I had to wake up early for training and so nothing was going to stop me falling asleep that night.

Nothing. Except maybe the odd ghost or two. Because a little while after I'd dropped off, I was woken up by the sound of footsteps outside my door. It was really loud and so I called downstairs to the front desk to tell them someone was making a racket and could they have a word with them.

A member of staff came up to my floor to see what was going on, knocked at my door and said, 'Miss, I'm sorry but there's nobody there.' By this time, the noises had gotten louder and I could hear constant whispering but I couldn't make out what was being said or exactly where the noise was coming from. The receptionist probably thought I had a screw loose or something and I didn't want to call them up again so I tried to get back to sleep.

It was then that I noticed the remote control for the TV, which had been next to the bed, was on the floor across the other side of the room. Not only that, the two books I'd been reading were scattered away from the bedside table where I'd left them. I was freaking out by this time – the whispering was still there and the temperature of the room had dropped to the point where I could see my breath as I exhaled. In the end, I must have dropped off to sleep from sheer exhaustion but in the morning I demanded a different room, obviously. I saw Joey Essex over breakfast and he'd had a similar experience. He was going nuts – luckily for him he was in a room with a mate of his so it wasn't so bad but at least he had a witness to it happening. I was relieved; it meant I wasn't going loopy, that this place had something going on.

The hotel staff agreed to move both of us to new rooms without any fuss, they were clearly ahead of the game – there must have been constant complaints about those rooms. The hotel had a modern wing built onto it and this was fine, no spooks in there, thankfully. It had been a terrible night and for the second time in my life it confirmed for me: I do not like ghosts, I don't want them, I don't find them amusing and I don't care what people say: they exist!

The *Splash!* torture continued. People were getting injured all over the place but there was a sort of 'we're all in this together' mentality, which kept us grinning through the pain. Or maybe we were grimacing. Anyway, it was quite an ordeal.

On the evening of Saturday 5th January 2013, the first episode went out. It was perfect family viewing time. It was presented by Gabby Logan and Vernon Kay and there was a judging panel who decided who would go through to the next round. This was combined with voting from the public. I was so nervous I actually puked before I went out to the pool. I managed a one-and-a-half somersault tuck from the three-metre spring-board. I was so proud of myself; for someone scared of heights and not a natural diver, I was thrilled.

The judges said I was: 'oozing guts and determination. The dive was great... your coordination was spot on.' I was second on the leaderboard at that point and it was a very proud moment. One of the Olympic diving trainers said if I'd have started training when I was young, I could have made it as a pro-swimmer. He was probably feeding me a load of rubbish but it made me feel good. The show may have gotten a lot of flak for being trashy but the viewing figures were good enough that it was commissioned for a second season, and for the people who took part, it really was tough and I definitely faced up to my height demons.

There were no egos on show at all because we were all beaten up so badly by the training, we were all nervous and hurting and, as a result, we all looked after each other. 'We know how hard this dive is for you but you can do it,' we'd say to each other, and it was a great experience.

Boy was I exhausted after the training though. I mean, really earth-shatteringly tired. I thought I was coming down with something because I ached all over, even my boobs hurt. Hmm. And my period was late. Double hmm.

I'd not had a period throughout my training for *Splash!* which hadn't really registered; I thought that because I'd been in the gym so much and then working so hard, maybe I'd skipped for that reason. Apart from anything else, Ty and I had probably been intimate no more than twice in the past few weeks, I was so beaten up and tired by the show. I told my mom and she said, 'Cap, you need to go and get a pregnancy test.'

What mom didn't know was that we'd stopped using contraception because we didn't think pregnancy was on the cards. We had two little babies on the way with our carrier and I'd relaxed. Pregnancy wasn't going to happen for me and so I had nothing to worry about any more…

I really didn't think that there was the slightest chance I could be expecting a baby but I took the test and, sure enough, that little blue line appeared immediately. It was clear as a bell – I was pregnant!

Can you imagine how I felt? Emotional doesn't quite cover it. It was almost too much to deal with, but mainly at this point, I couldn't believe it. So I decided to do about ten more tests. I downed a litre of water and just sat on the loo doing one test after another and each and every test came back positive. To say I was in shock would be an understatement. 'Holy smokes, I'm pregnant,' I believe is what I said, out loud, in my bathroom.

I staggered to the phone in a daze and called Ty. 'Are you sitting down? I have something important to tell you… I'm pregnant.' Ty was really stuck for words. He tried to say something but nothing came out. The phone went dead and he turned up at home about half an hour later, wanting to see each of those pregnancy tests for himself.

I knew it was amazing, unbelievable, a miracle – but at the same time I was completely aware of the many reasons this might not yet work out. Ty's reaction was, 'Oh fuck, I'm having three kids,' or words to that effect – minus the 'F' word. That's what I would say, not Ty.

Because we'd hardly had sex in the past few weeks, we could pinpoint the conception date quite easily and it meant that this baby (or babies – oh my god, what if it were twins?) would be born about a month after our carrier gave birth.

We didn't breathe a word to anyone but I called up the Chelsea and Westminster to see if they'd see me. They remembered me from the time I'd miscarried the twins and were amazing. They didn't have to give me a scan – it's not NHS policy without a referral – but they did. I saw the exact same lady who'd nursed me before and they were so accommodating. The last time I'd been in it had been a day and a half of horror for me. They were so kind because they'd seen what I'd gone through last time.

As the sonographer scanned for a fetus we held our breaths. 'It's very early on in the pregnancy, probably about four weeks, but everything seems to be fine so far,' she said. I couldn't believe it. Ty squeezed my hand and I tried hard to hold back tears. All the horror of the last miscarriage couldn't be wiped away with a single scan but it went a long way towards giving both of us hope. How this pregnancy could happen after weeks of arduous training I have no idea and no expert has ever come up with a reason why or how. It really was a miracle.

Chapter 15

When Two Become Four

Of course, there was the small matter of how to break it to Tina, and I'd test the lines out myself when I was at home with Ty. I'd pretend to be on the phone to her and I'd say, 'How does this sound: "So, we're not sure how it's happened but I seem to be pregnant…"?' Nope. Too flippant. 'How about, "We have something to tell you, it's a miracle – I'm pregnant – but please don't worry, we desperately want all three children and this doesn't change anything."' But nothing sounded right. It sounded weird, even to my ears. What if she thought we'd done it on purpose, in order to have an 'instant' family? So many concerns and no one to guide us on this one; we were alone. It's not exactly a typical situation, is it?

Before we could go any further and act on our thoughts, something really traumatic happened. I started to bleed. By this time I was still only about six weeks pregnant and was just getting used to the idea of having a child I would carry myself and give birth to. I don't know if I quite believed it would happen but maybe I'd allowed myself to think those thoughts and start to picture myself with two newborns. And now it was going to be over before it ever really began – or so I thought at that moment.

Ty and I were supposed to be going out to see one of his friends when it happened and as I lay there feeling scared and not wanting to move at all, the phone rang. It was my doctor's office in America with even worse news: our carrier had lost one of the babies and they were about to scan her to find out what was going on and to make sure the other embryo was still OK. We would discover later we'd lost a baby girl.

Within half an hour we had gone from having three babies on the way to potentially having one. I sat there and sobbed my heart out. This whole thing was such torture and it felt so unfair. After everything we'd been through and now this – I felt like my heart was breaking. I called the hospital and begged them to see me – as it was, they'd seen me far more frequently than was usual but they knew how petrified I was of losing this baby after what had happened last time.

They agreed. I went in, lay down on the bed and held my breath. I sensed they were almost as nervous as I was. God knows how I'd react if anything was wrong, so they were probably feeling a little anxious about that. I was so damn emotional. I waited for what seemed like forever. I wanted to scream with frustration, although I didn't have the breath to scream; I was holding it in too much.

After a moment, the sonographer who was scanning me said with a little smile on her face:

'We have a heartbeat!' and she had a note of triumph in her voice. I was so happy, and they were very sympathetic this time around. I felt as though they were on this journey with me.

I sat in that tiny room and I prayed and thanked whoever it is out there for giving me this chance. I was so appreciative. Throughout this process I'd become more and more aware of the pain and challenges of becoming a mother for some people. I'd always assumed my body would deliver the goods, no problem. When I'd gone into this process I'd had no idea of what women (and their partners) go through to have a child, and the sense of desolation it can bring. But at that moment, I was full of hope and joy and I never wanted to let that feeling go.

I asked her if she would give me a moment, a flood of tears rolled down my face. Everything was OK, I had two healthy babies.

The doctor explained that in the early weeks of pregnancy there can be some bleeding as the embryo embeds itself into the uterus or occasionally, it can happen around the time your period would be due.

Our other baby, the son Tina was carrying, was also fine and developing well. We didn't know why we'd lost one of the babies and, in a way, didn't want to dwell on it. It had to be all about the future and the two children we knew we had. Of course this meant that I was totally paranoid about losing the baby I was carrying and I did everything in my power to keep healthy. Because of the tests we'd had before insemination, we already knew our son Tina was carrying would be healthy.

By this time, I think the girls in my office at By Caprice knew what was going on but they were terribly English about it and no one asked outright!

But I kind of took a little bit of a back seat for a while and trusted them to get on with running things. This is not something that comes naturally to me at all, but my baby had to be my priority. I would do anything and everything I could to make sure my babies would carry to full-term. The hospital were so great, they didn't seem to mind my turning up more regularly than I was meant to (I mean, every week!) for a scan because they'd seen the truly horrible time I'd had during my miscarriage. I had to gear myself up for a bad outcome and I couldn't let myself get too excited for the baby I was carrying; not yet anyway.

If I'd have lost this baby at this stage – even though I wasn't far into the pregnancy – I'm not sure I'd have been able to cope without spiralling deep down into the depths of despair. For now, at least, I could enjoy the moment, but I wasn't about to take any of it for granted.

I did wrap myself up in cotton wool for a while and Ty must have felt he was living with some kind of nun! I slept as much as I could, I didn't go out more than I needed to, I stopped working out and watched a lot of movies instead. I ate the healthiest organic food, took all my antenatal vitamins and laid low.

We were in Florida for the Easter/Passover break and by now my boobs were feeling tender and they were growing. I'd gone from a 34C to a 34DD. My stomach no longer looked like I'd eaten four big bowls of pasta, it actually looked like I was in the early stages of pregnancy. I'd expressed my concern to Ty on this trip, that if I were photographed during this break before Tina had heard it from me, she would understandably feel very hurt and probably worried.

And of course this is exactly what happened – I was photographed on the beach and the next thing was, I was splashed all over the cover of *Closer* magazine.

Vickie called me and said, 'Cap, we have a situation. There are some pictures of you in a bikini on the cover of *Closer* magazine and they say you're pregnant. I'm getting a lot of calls about it.' I told her to say nothing and that I would call her back. I ran downstairs to tell Ty what had happened – It was now or never: I had to tell Tina, even though it was still quite early days.

She knew I had quite a high profile in the UK and all it would take would be a few clicks of the mouse to discover my secret.

We'd wanted to wait as long as possible to tell anyone, after all; so much could go wrong – and had gone wrong. Ty and I were still almost in a state of disbelief ourselves about the whole thing. 'Could it be that this pregnancy will actually work?' I would say most days to Ty.

Before talking to Tina I decided to call my IVF doctor in the States to tell him the news. I was on my mobile in my room, looking out at the sea. I asked the receptionist to please get my doctor as I had some urgent news to tell him. Of course I was being dramatic to make sure he took my call immediately.

He picked up the phone and asked if everything was all right. I said: 'Yes, but I have something to tell you. I'm pregnant.'

He said, 'Yes, I know you're having a child via a carrier,' but I said, 'No, you don't understand, I'm pregnant.' There was what felt like a full two minutes of dead silence. In the end I said: 'Hello! Doc, are you still there?'

'Yes, Cap, and I'm delighted, but I have to tell you, in my 25 years' experience something like this has never happened. I wish I could give you some medical reason as to how this has come about but all I can say is, this is a miracle.'

Maybe it was something to do with the fact I was relaxed and not even dreaming of falling pregnant when it happened, but this still doesn't explain why my uterus could suddenly hold onto an embryo, feed it, nourish it and retain it for a full pregnancy. I hadn't done anything different this time around; that's why it was such a miracle and why no one – within reason – should give up hope of having a child.

With my doctor fully in the picture it was time. I had to call Tina. 'I hope you're sitting down because I have to tell you something and it's something I was *not* anticipating.'

'I think I know. You're pregnant, aren't you?' said Tina. Somehow she'd just guessed. Maybe she had been studying some of those paparazzi pictures on the internet and drawn her own conclusions but anyhow, now she knew and she was wonderful about it.

'I suspected but I knew you would want to tell me in your own time,' she admitted to me. Sure enough she'd seen the pictures. She thought maybe I was faking it! She said to me: 'I thought maybe you were trying to tell people you were pregnant and you weren't going to reveal the fact you used a carrier for the pregnancy.'

I told her: 'If you see anything that worries you again, just call me, even if it's something bad that you're thinking, you gotta tell me because I'll always be honest about it. I really didn't want to worry you. You're carrying my child and for that I am eternally grateful.'

Most of all, I really didn't want her to think I was a just another celebrity paying for someone to have my baby, so it didn't wreck my body. This has definitely been the case in Hollywood circles for a while now but for me, being pregnant and feeling the baby kick and wriggle inside of me and for me to experience getting bigger and fatter every day was all part of the thrill of being pregnant, something vital and magical I really didn't want to miss out on.

I explained to her that Ty and I had wanted to wait for as long as possible to tell anyone because of everything we'd gone through. She is such a lovely lady she said: 'I'm so happy for you, you're having two kids now and we have each other to support during this special time.'

From that moment on, we shared our pregnancies with each other and she was such a wonderful help to me because she'd gone through having her babies before and knew what to expect. We would call each other and I'd say, 'How about this, I think I felt a kick, is it too early?' and she'd say, 'I'm a little bit tired today, pregnancy sure can make you feel emotional,' and I'd agree because actually, my hormones were all over the place, too.

I'm someone who's very used to feeling in control and throughout my pregnancy I was very emotional. If someone so much as crushed a fly I'd feel tears pricking at my eyes. For a while, I couldn't control anything and I was worried I'd turn into someone who couldn't keep themselves together. I'm usually very business-like in the way I deal with people but it wasn't until about four months after the birth that I finally felt 'myself' again. It was a relief, I can tell you! It's probably the one area of the pregnancy I didn't enjoy too much.

And so our pregnancies carried on, with my babies growing inside of us, and for a while, everything was peaceful. I felt much less tired as the weeks went by and I was healthy and hungry! I ate everything in sight and didn't care about getting bigger and fatter – the way I felt about this was that my babies would need all the nourishment I could give them!

I was still as focused as I possibly could be with By Caprice, despite all that was going on with my babies – and in our spare time, Ty and I enjoyed our time together. He had broken the news of the babies to his children, whom we were seeing every weekend, and though of course it had been a shock to them, they seemed to be gradually getting used to the idea.

This book isn't the place to talk about someone else's children, but Ty's three kids are wonderful and I love them very much. I love the way they've embraced their new brothers. It was always my dream to have a big, happy family and I'm so fortunate to have just that.

Being pregnant and running a multi-national business isn't easy, as anyone who's been through it will tell you. I delegated a lot to my team so I didn't have to travel very much, and made sure the business was in good shape for me to try and take a step back when the babies were born. As you'll probably have realised, By Caprice had been my 'baby' up until now and so it certainly didn't come easily to hand over anything to anyone else, but it was in a good place. On the back of the success of using Amy Childs we'd decided to sign up another hot new TV name, this time, *TOWIE*'s Lucy Mecklenburgh, and as well as using other models I also began to expand my range.

There are other benefits to becoming a mom: the empathy you have for women's ever-changing bodies. The body you go into pregnancy with is not the one you come out with, no matter how careful you are, and it has given me a real appreciation for the different shapes and sizes we women come in.

I started to think more about this and to develop ideas for the larger cup sizes. I found a new creative energy – I've heard this is quite common in pregnancy and for me, it kicked in at around the five-month mark. I felt great, I looked healthy and I'd started to get that pregnancy glow at last! Not everything went according to plan though.

When Tina was about five months pregnant she fell ill with a high temperature that just wouldn't go down. She ended up in hospital with some kind of infection and they pumped her full of antibiotics, which of course really scared me. The earlier in a pregnancy antibiotics are taken, the more likely the risk of damage to the baby and this was uppermost in my mind.

I know now that some antibiotics are considered safe for a fetus to be exposed to but at that time, apart from being concerned for my carrier, Tina, it was my baby who was at risk, too. After all the checks we'd made about how Tina was living and eating, to have her catch an infection we could do nothing about was very hard to bear.

Tina was so ill and we were all so worried, we were calling every couple of hours but they never did get to the bottom of whatever the infection was and after a couple of days she was allowed home. And then the strangest thing happened. When I was exactly the same number of weeks pregnant, I fell ill with almost exactly the same symptoms. I was in a car, on my way home from doing a TV interview when I started to feel full of aches and pains and really nauseous – but at the same time I was hot all over.

I sat on my sofa and thought, this is not right, I don't feel good at all. Ty was trying to reassure me but my mom, on the other hand, was on the phone saying, 'Get yourself to the doctor now, you can't mess about, you're pregnant!' By this stage I could barely stand and within hours I'd been admitted to hospital and put on a drip. I was hallucinating because they couldn't get my temperature down – it had reached 40°C. I have very hazy memories of what was going on at this point as I was vomiting and had become dangerously dehydrated. The nurse kept trying to keep me awake as she thought she was going to lose me – she thought if my blood pressure continued to drop I could have died. She called Emergency and I was being packed up to go to intensive care (the staff told me all this afterwards).

'How's my daughter, what are you giving her? Will she be OK? How's the baby?' Mom was demanding down the phone. London feels like a very long way from LA when your pregnant daughter is in hospital. Ty was travelling and so I was on my own but I was too ill to worry about that. And then suddenly my blood pressure started to stabilise and finally, by the next morning, my temperature also dropped back to normal.

After a few hours I was through the worst of it, thank god. But then the nurse came in and wanted to check on the baby. I had a strap put around my stomach whilst they used the monitor on me and they started to use the scanner to find the baby and listen to the heartbeat.

After a few minutes I started to worry. 'What's the matter? Why do you have that look on your face?'

But the doctor wouldn't look at me, she just kept working the scanner backwards and forwards and looking at the monitor. I could feel panic rising after five minutes of this. 'Why aren't you telling me what's going on? What's the problem?' I tried not to get hysterical but her silence and her serious expression were really frightening me.

Finally, her face relaxed. She found the heartbeat and a smile appeared. 'Don't worry, I have it now,' she said. The relief in the room was palpable. I was still pregnant, my baby was fine – that was all I needed to know.

I'd publicly announced my pregnancy at the beginning of May when I was about five months pregnant – we'd managed to keep it quiet for that long somehow, probably because I'd not been to any events in months.

And so, people knew I was pregnant but they didn't know the whole story – how in the hell was I going to tackle talking about my surrogate? It was only a matter of time before someone found out the truth.

On the one hand this was all so private, I really wanted Ty and me to go through both pregnancies without any media attention. On the other hand, when you're in the public eye you realise early on that people feel they have a right to know what's going on in your private life, especially if it is a good

215

story. I was used to it, Ty wasn't, and of course it took a while for him to understand why we would need to share some information.

There were lots of approaches from magazines and TV for talking about my pregnancy in more depth but at that point I'd said all I wanted to say, which was just to confirm my pregnancy. Once the story was out though, it was fabulous to be able to relax and not have to hide my growing bump. There's a picture of Ty and me at a wonderful ball that month called the Caldwell Children's Charity Butterfly Ball. It was the first official 'outing' of my baby bump and it was so wonderful to be able to talk freely about my pregnancy at last!

What wasn't so great was the looming story about our gestational carrier, which we knew was a big story if any media got hold of it. We'd talked about how to break the story but our hands were forced when, in very early June, Vickie took a call from *The Sun*. They told her they knew from a reliable source that I was having a baby via a surrogate and that they were going to run the story even if I didn't confirm it.

I was completely thrown by this because I'd kept things very quiet about my carrier; I wanted to protect my unborn children more than my own life. I certainly didn't want people digging around trying to find out who this lady was and disrupting her family as well as compromising our privacy. This was one of the reasons I'd worked with an agency in the US rather than the UK. I hated the idea that people would make judgements about my carrier or about Ty and me and what we'd done. We'd been through so much to have these babies; I was feeling fragile and very protective and wanted to have some control over the news.

We had a big decision to make: if the story hit the press and was uncorroborated by Ty and me, it may be slanderous and very hurtful. We would also have no control at all – yes, we could sue them but what good would it do? We might get an apology on page 590 but it would be too late: the story would be repeated over and over, amplified by other papers and magazines and websites and we couldn't sue everyone. I knew from past experience this tactic just didn't work.

My mom said: 'I am sick to death of these lies being printed about you and you not defending yourself. You have to stand up and own the story yourself this time.' We knew – Ty, Mom, Vickie and me – that keeping quiet was not going to make the story go away. The only real reason I was holding off was because I hated the idea people would attack me or, far worse, attack my children – who weren't even born yet!

But I had to see the bigger picture. True, I was scared I would be torn to pieces by people saying, 'Why didn't she just adopt?' or, 'It's her fault for leaving it too late.'

So, I took a deep breath and said: 'OK, let's do this. We'll talk to *The Sun* in-depth and tell them everything that's happened.' I didn't want to leave anything out. I didn't want anyone crawling out of the woodwork with more to tell because I'd not told the whole truth from the start. This was to be the whole, unadulterated story.

'Caprice to have two babies in four weeks', said *The Sun*'s headline a few weeks later. A little misleading but, hey, it's a tricky story to get across, I guess.

The story was published and, whoosh! It was as if someone lit the blue touch paper and the story took on a life of its own.

My manager's phone was ringing off the hook, as was mine. We had requests for interviews from all the major TV companies, newspapers and magazines as well as the radio stations, here and in the US. All of a sudden it was a major story. *The Sun* had split it into two parts: a front cover one day and then a few days later it was a few pages inside, too. The *Daily Mail* pretty much repeated the story on their front page after *The Sun* – unheard of!

I couldn't bear to read it. I remember handing it over to Ty without looking and saying: 'You read it. What have they said, are they tearing us apart?' After a few minutes, when I'd finally allowed him to go through it he looked up and said: 'It's very nice. You have nothing to worry about.' That was good news, but oh god, my stress levels were through the roof at this point.

Then I braced myself to look at the *Mail Online*. Anyone in the public eye dreads reading the public's comments under their picture – they're lying if they say they don't – and I was petrified. They usually kick things off about me by saying, 'She's not 41... she's 85' or words to that effect. And so, with great trepidation, I peered at the comments, virtually through my fingers.

'Hey, they're being really nice!' I was astonished! Everyone was so kind and understanding and compassionate. I felt very emotional (as usual in this pregnancy) reading through the comments.

Vickie was being inundated with requests for interviews, which I wasn't going to do. The whole point of *The Sun's* piece was to get the correct story out there and not the story an unknown parasite sold to make a few pounds. Some people have no shame or consideration. I hope you don't mind me going on a little rant right now, but there is one side of being in the public eye that is a constant let-down. You can't really trust anyone, at least, sadly, this is how I feel after 20 years of being a public figure.

I did agree to do one TV interview: *This Morning* with Philip Schofield and Holly Willoughby. It was an atmosphere I felt comfortable in, with people I could trust.

Again, I felt I wanted to do one TV interview to get the story straight, the way I wanted it to be heard and I'm so glad we did it this way.

From that moment on, it felt like I had a huge wave of emotional support behind me – the British public were lovely to me – I felt so much affection from people it confirmed what I'd felt for many years: I'm an honorary Brit. I might have a US passport and I'm proud to be American, but I'm also proud to feel British. I feel this country has adopted me and the all-American Valley Girl who arrived here back in 1996 has become a fully-fledged English Rose ... Well, kind of.

Chapter 16

Miracles can Happen

Of course I had a baby shower! Thrown for me by my friend Wanda, who lives in Hawaii and whom I've known forever.

It was fabulous. Wanda invited 40 of my friends from the past 18 years in the UK and we all sat around and gossiped and they gave me such beautiful gifts. Having a baby was suddenly very real; here was a tiny Babygro, there were teensy cute booties and all of these things would soon actually be on my babies! Everyone was so happy for Ty and me and as I looked around the room at all these women whom I love so much, I realised how much my life had changed.

Even without babies in the picture, I'd become someone who had a close network of supportive girlfriends. I had friends from all walks of life – from the entertainment business, socialites, and regular 9-5 people who weren't in the public eye – and it was so special. I was inundated with offers from magazines to come along and take pictures but I really wanted this to be a private party.

The cake was fabulous and the beautiful gifts I was given took up about a quarter of my living room when I finally got them all home! I did a little speech and told everyone how grateful I was that they'd taken a day off in the middle of the week to come to my baby shower and shown me such love and support over the years. I cannot believe how important these girls have become to me and what a girl's girl I've become! It was such a great moment for me to share that time with my friends.

Later on that day, Ty and I headed off to the incredibly glam Serpentine summer party. We were surrounded by society's best, from the Jaggers to Sarah Jessica Parker and Princess Beatrice – it was a perfect day from start to finish.

Everything was coming together, and some days I had to pinch myself.

I mean, I still had to pack up everything ready for the flight to LA. I also had to pack my entire rented house and put everything into storage as when we got back to London I would have my two new baby boys. We had just found a house – well, a wreck – we wanted to convert into our new home. It was going to take a lot of work to transform the building, but we knew it had enormous potential.

My business was firing on all cylinders. We were about to shoot our next campaign with Lucy Mecklenburgh – so there was a lot to cram in over the last few weeks before my babies were born. We knew by this time we were having boys and we'd discussed names but we weren't quite in agreement yet on them.

I could feel my stress levels rising, though I tried hard to take it easy. But the pressure was building as I knew I'd be taking time out after the birth. I wasn't planning on taking long off, probably a few months at this stage (hmm, it didn't quite work out that way!) but I still felt I needed to cross all the t's and dot all the i's before signing off for a while.

I was at my desk, head in the world of finance and lingerie when my mobile phone rang. It was Tina.

'Hi Cap, I don't want to worry you but I'm dilating – it means the baby might not be as far off being born as we thought. It's unpredictable – it could be three weeks or it could be tomorrow but I'd feel more comfortable if you were here.'

When a baby is born, the cervix dilates – or opens – first of all up to 5cm and from then on, with the pressure of the baby pushing down on the birth canal, it will open to 10cm to allow the baby to be born. But I thought that once you started to dilate that meant you were going to give birth straight away and so I freaked out and jumped on the first flight I could get. I thought, 'I'm going to have my first child right now', but thankfully it wasn't quite what I anticipated.

Because my carrier had given birth four times before, she had the experience to know what was happening and to know that it was hard to tell what dilation might mean. Even so, I went into a little bit of a tailspin. It was all happening too fast, too early! I really wasn't ready at all. I had my mom help me with sorting out the house in LA – I wanted it to be just perfect for when the boys were born. In between juggling calls from solicitors, I was trying to pack all we would need for LA and arrange a lingerie campaign – all on top of moving out of our current home. I thought my head was about to explode. So much for taking it easy in the last weeks of pregnancy! All those weeks I'd been so careful at the beginning and I ended up tearing around in the last days.

But it was all happening about three weeks earlier than expected and so I ended up throwing things into boxes and shoving them in storage. It was all a mess but it had to be done before we left. Our home in Notting Hill wouldn't be our home when we brought the boys back to the UK later in the year – we'd be living in our amazing new place. Finally, after a year of continual negotiations over costs and design issues, our dream house would be finished.

I asked Becky, who does my PR how I was behaving then and she said, 'Because we knew your carrier was already dilating, and you were really keen to fly out to the States, it was touch and go that day as to whether you could actually make the shoot. We really thought you'd be on a plane somewhere over the Atlantic, but, Cap, you were as professional and as in control as you always are. Watching as you showed Lucy different poses at eight months pregnant was kind of interesting, though!'

We managed to get through all the shots with Lucy Mecklenburgh in one day – that was an entire swimwear and lingerie range in a ten-hour stretch. Lucy's manager was great, pulling the photo shoot forwards to help us out, and she did a fantastic job. Lucy looked fabulous: she's curvy and feminine with a super-hot body but she's also very beautiful. She encompassed everything my brand is about: sexy, current, stylish – but still retaining a little bit of the girl-next-door. I loved her. That campaign ended up being huge when it launched in November – one of our biggest ever and it was all done under such pressure, too!

Meanwhile, the doctors in LA were telling Ty and me to stick to our original flight date: 'There's no rush to get here, she's not going to give birth for quite a while yet,' they reassured us. It wasn't what our carrier was saying.

'Cap, I just have this feeling that you need to come soon,' she said.

'Believe me, honey, I'm on it, I'll be there,' I told her and it was true. I went into overdrive with everything, maybe this is the so-called nesting instinct women allegedly have because somehow I managed to get on that plane almost a month earlier than I'd first intended. Wow, the feeling of blissful relief I felt when I made that flight was unbelievable!

After the 11-hour flight, we landed in LA to beautiful weather. It was great to be able to head to my house and just relax at last. I would still be emailing and following the business daily but I felt I had permission now to enjoy some time off before my babies were born.

And of course, it was time to meet Tina! We had exchanged lots of photos and talked constantly but we'd never met face to face and then was the moment.

I went to the hospital to meet her as she had a check-up with the doctor and as the door opened I went straight to her and gave her a massive cuddle. We both hugged each other for ages, took lots of pictures together to show our children when they were older, and really enjoyed the moment. She is such a wonderful person, so warm and caring, I feel Ty and I have been utterly blessed to find her. I couldn't have wished for a better person to carry my child.

Thankfully we had a little bit of breathing space as there were no signs of labour for the next couple of weeks.

Every day I would wake up nervous and full of excitement for what lay ahead. I'd heard that the work on our new home had started and although it was frustrating not being there to oversee it, I had to let go for the first time in my life.

'Sit down, relax, have a swim, get a pedicure,' my mom would say to me.

Already I felt a shift in my relationship with Mom. Things felt calmer between us than they'd felt in a long time. We'd always had a good relationship, but these last couple of years had brought us ever closer. Mom had been so involved with and supportive of the IVF and surrogacy process. She'd always been so busy with her business but she was making time for me and what she knew was a huge deal in my life, and that meant so much to me.

Tina called me early one morning: 'I think I might be in labour, so I'll just go to the hospital and get checked in,' she said. She was so unbelievably calm. I, of course, had been waiting for the news ever since we'd arrived and I was so excited and nervous. I couldn't wait to get to the hospital.

Ty and I packed a few things in a bag, looked at each other and I said, 'This is it, we're about to become parents together.' We took a deep breath, and climbed into our car.

I'd thought that Tina's labour might be quite quick because she'd had four children already, but she explained each labour had been different so we really didn't know what to expect. In the event, it went pretty slowly. When she arrived at the hospital she was 4cm dilated (the cervix needs to be 10cm dilated to actually give birth) and it took forever to get to 7cm. Tina said it was much longer than normal; the day dragged on and on… but in fact we had so much fun!

My mom was there, and Tina's husband, along with Ty and me. We were laughing and chatting away.

It was baking hot outside and at eight months pregnant I spent my life trying to cool down, so the best thing was that Tina's hospital room was freezing. It was wonderful for me! Not for everyone else, though. They were all sitting there with their teeth chattering, cuddled up in five blankets whilst I was there in a vest, loving the cold air!

The hospital had given Tina her own room – and they gave one to us as well. By midnight we were really tired and Tina insisted I went for a rest. (Me! She was the one in labour!) She promised to call us when the time came.

While Ty and I went off to sleep, Tina's husband went to the cafeteria to get something to eat and so Tina was left alone with my mom and the nurse for a while. After about half an hour, my mom ran into the room screaming, 'She's having the baby she's having the baby!' – it was time. Tina was ready to push! Her husband couldn't be reached though; there was no phone signal in the café but she really needed him there and so there was this last minute flurry of activity whilst we tried to find him. And then, all of a sudden he walked into the room with a quesadilla in his hand. He saw Ty and me holding Tina's hand and he was over to her in a flash.

I was trying to help Tina to breathe through the pain and at the same time I kept my eye on the doctor as she smiled at me reassuringly.

Tina was so amazing, she warned me that just before starting to push, her body would shake and that this was completely normal; throughout this whole thing she was reassuring me, even though she was the one giving birth to my son. She knew I was worried about going through labour for the first time and she wanted me to be prepared rather than scared. Soon after this, she asked for a sheet to be set up to give her some privacy – this meant Ty and I were holding her hand but we couldn't see very much.

The doctor smiled at me and said: 'He's coming…' Tina took a deep breath, determined and so strong at that moment – and she pushed once and then just one more time and that was it. A little after 12am the baby, my baby, was born.

Within seconds, I'd cut the umbilical cord but I was sobbing so hard I could barely see what I was doing. The doctor picked up my baby and handed him to me.

I've never felt such a closeness with anyone in my life, I took all my clothes off from my waist up, totally oblivious to everyone else in the room, and when my son hit my naked skin he immediately stopped crying. I just wanted him to be able to smell his mommy straight away. He looked at me and I at him. At that point everyone in the room had tears streaming down their faces. I can't describe in words the immense feeling of love, devotion, hope and appreciation for this moment. Everyone in the room felt it, including the nurse who'd just arrived at work 40 minutes prior; it was magic.

'I wish I had a picture of this moment,' Tina said, and then realised: 'I'm done! I can take the pictures!'

My mom was designated photographer but she was doing a crap job because she was too busy crying and so Tina decided that she needed to take over. Oh my gosh, she has just given birth to my son and she's taking on the role of photographer? You can't even write this sort of stuff in a movie. So there Tina was, snapping away with her mobile phone.

She said she felt completely fine and she wanted to make sure Ty and I had plenty of private time with our baby. She said she knew from her own experience how important it was to have this quiet time and how special it was.

And so we sat with him, just gazing at his tiny, beautiful face, looking at this little miracle we thought we'd never be able to have, and it was so wonderful – even now I find it hard putting it into words. Everything – from the doctors to how wonderful Tina was – had made it the best day of my life. I wouldn't let our baby go, I just held onto him for hours and the connection I had with him was so intense, it was beyond a bond. I looked at him and I could see such a family resemblance. And I could see how much he looked like the scans we'd seen of him. Ty laughed at me and said I was a complete nutcase because to him our son's face in the scan looked like mush. But my mom and I could clearly see a family resemblance – but maybe this is just a mommy thing.

I'd asked Tina if she'd use a breast pump so I could feed my son the all-important colostrum. This is the highly nutritious first milk, which contains all kinds of antibodies and it's really important babies have this to help protect against infection. It's produced in that last few weeks of pregnancy and I really wanted my first-born to have it. We stayed overnight and made sure the next day that he was able to feed OK and then we were allowed to take him home.

I was really worried for Tina. She'd never given birth to a child and had to give it away immediately and although she'd assured us all the way through the pregnancy that she was happy to do it, there was still that worry she'd find it terribly traumatic. After all, she'd carried the baby, her hormones might be firing off all over the place and she was probably exhausted from giving birth.

But the wonderful, incredible thing was, Tina seemed completely fine. She told me when she left the hospital, she felt as though she'd been in for some other, minor procedure, certainly not having just given birth!

I totally take my hat off to her, to go through this for someone and to come out of it unscathed in any way is pretty remarkable. Tina and her family are now part of our family. Whenever we're in the States we all meet up. My boys know her as Auntie Tina and my children love their 'cousins', Tina's four children. We're always sending each other pictures. The fact that she's decided to go for a second surrogate pregnancy doesn't surprise me at all: she told me she'd loved the experience and that seeing the joy on our faces at the birth made it all worthwhile. As I've said many times, I can never thank her enough for what she did for us.

The birth of my second son was a very different experience. The doc had warned me that the umbilical cord was around my baby's neck and as far as I was concerned, this was a very good reason to go straight for a Caesarean section. 'After all we've been through, I'm not risking anything,' I told my doc. 'I'm not taking any chances whatsoever.' Whilst someone else who'd had no problems at all might have risked it, I wasn't that person. I wanted my baby in my arms in the safest way possible and so the doctor agreed.

I was on the phone to my office in London, with my first-born son cuddled up against me when it happened. I got a shot of pain, like the worst kind of period pain imaginable and as it coursed through my body I knew: I was in labour.

I tried hard not to panic and I carried on going through with my phone call. We were discussing the latest collection, which was due to go out soon in a few weeks but there it was again: the pain.

I asked my mom to hold my son for a second. She took one look at me and said, 'Cap, I think you're in labour. We need to call the hospital.' I felt really upset. 'This isn't meant to happen, I'm booked in for the Caesarean and I'm only just within my due date. I'm sure it's a false alarm,' I said, looking to her for reassurance. None was forthcoming, unfortunately. She took charge and it wasn't long before Ty and I were on our way to hospital with Mom at home with my baby. This couldn't be happening now, I wasn't ready, but the nurse confirmed it when I was examined: I was dilating and I was officially in labour. Because I was due to have a Caesarean, they acted pretty quickly and I was prepped for surgery within an hour of arriving at the hospital.

This time, the operating theatre was freezing again but I was the one shaking like a leaf, partly from fear, partly as the shock of what was happening to me kicked in. I was in a lot of pain but, again, I didn't want anything for the pain because it always makes me feel ill and so I had to wait until I was given anaesthetic into my spine to numb me from the chest down. I couldn't believe it: I thought I'd be knocked out completely for the operation but, once I'd had that jab in my spine that was it, the surgeon cracked on with the job – all to the tunes of the Rolling Stones!

There I was, lying on the bed, freezing to death with my teeth chattering, listening to my skin 'fry' as they cut me open, with a very disturbing scent of flesh in my nostrils.

At the same time, 'Brown Sugar' is blaring from the speakers and he's practically rocking out to the music there in front of me! They're a lot more laid back in America than they are in the UK. It was a bizarre feeling as I could feel my doctor's hand roaming around inside of me, but there was no pain. I'm sure it's like that with everyone, but it freaked me out.

Ty was beside me the whole time but as the procedure went on, he said I got paler and paler. After a few minutes I said, 'Where's my baby?' and he said, 'I can't find him yet,' and carried on with the rummaging. Finally, after what seemed like hours but was probably only a few minutes, the rummaging stopped and they pulled out my beautiful son.

It certainly wasn't the nurturing, joyful experience I'd had the first time around; this felt much more like I was part of a machine, although a very well-run machine. I'm sure thousands of women go through this every day but I think because it was so recent that I'd had such a positive experience, it really seemed to highlight the differences to me. Still, the most important thing was that I had another perfect, healthy son.

Of course with a Caesarean you can't immediately hold your baby because you need to be sewn up. So I wasn't given my baby straight away but I could hear him crying, which was a relief. I knew he was OK. The doc, meanwhile, said: 'I'm just going to zip you up now,' which somehow just seemed kind of inappropriate in the middle of something so momentous. And the stitching seemed to go on and on forever, with layer and layer of stitches being done. The baby was being weighed and Ty had cut the umbilical cord and I was desperate to see my second-born son. I was taken into the recovery room and I felt so sick. I was still absolutely freezing too.

I think it was about two hours before I actually got to hold my baby and that was the longest two hours of my entire life. I wanted to see him, I missed him, but I'd just come out of surgery and so I needed looking after. I don't know if the process is exactly the same in the UK but for me, if I had no potential complications, I would definitely opt for a natural birth.

What was also torture was that they wouldn't allow my first-born son into the hospital to sleep with me, and this was incredibly painful. He was only a few weeks old and we'd not been apart at all yet. I was tearful and upset and just wanted to take my baby home and see my first-born for a cuddle too. I slept very little those first few days. My son would lie on my chest in the hospital and we'd both fall asleep fitfully on and off throughout the night as I was breastfeeding.

When I was allowed home, putting the boys next to each other on the bed, looking at these tiny little people we'd created, I was almost speechless with joy. We'd named them Jett and Jax and apart from close family and our carrier, no one knew which boy had been born first – and we intend to keep it that way as it's irrelevant; they're both biologically our boys.

But I was also completely exhausted. I wasn't sleeping very much because I was in pain from the operation. I didn't want to take painkillers because I was afraid of it entering the babies' bloodstreams as I was breastfeeding them both. The first month I didn't leave the house because I literally had one or both of my boys on the breast the whole time. I had a bit of a break between 12.30am and 4.30am but other than that they were both busy sucking the life out of me. After one month my nipples were like a war zone: raw and bleeding. But I resisted the pain and invested in nipple protectors

– the best investment when you're breastfeeding two raven-ous boys. I'm sure you're wondering if my first-born took to breastfeeding after a few weeks of being formula-fed and yes, he did! It was like a duck taking to water – he latched on im-mediately and never let it go. I had to pull him off after thirty minutes each time.

Breastfeeding might be natural but getting the right sit-ting position without giving yourself back pain and being comfortable when your breasts and nipples are killing is not easy. I'd employed a wonderful maternity nurse to help show me what to do. I was pretty clueless at this stage! She really helped me to learn how to feed them properly and try and get them into some sort of routine. But this was a new situ-ation for her, too. Two babies, just a few weeks apart, was a challenge. If you've had a baby, you'll know that they can change so much from one week to the next and almost from one day to the next, and so it was tough in the beginning.

After a few nights struggling to keep both babies fed prop-erly, my mom took one look at me and said, 'Cap, you're going to pass out if you don't get some rest.' She took the boys away and topped them up with formula milk through the night. I did pass out – into a very deep, dreamless, blissful sleep for a whole ten hours.

I was so sore those first few weeks, I had real trouble moving around and I found that really hard, as I'm usually constantly on the move. I'm not someone who enjoys being plonked down on the sofa and told to stay. I had to get used to taking it easy. I tried not to pick the boys up too much because I'd been warned it could cause a tear in my Caesarean scar, but it's impossible! There's these two beautiful munchkins and

234

all you want to do is constantly pick them up and cuddle them. And so I did end up with a little bit of an infection but I was fine – all I cared about were my boys.

These two beautiful babies were my miracles and I wanted to just savour this time we had together. Ty was with us a lot of the time but he had to work and so he was backwards and forwards between the US and the UK, but my mom was with me and she was such a great help and I appreciate the time and love she gave all of us.

After a few weeks I'd go out for a gentle walk and I'd come home to find one or the other baby asleep on mom's chest and they clearly adored her and she did them. She and I might have had our differences in the past and she could be quite tempestuous and dramatic sometimes – we're both Scorpios and sometimes we could have some pretty serious rows – but during this period and ever since, she became a solid, wonderful fixture in their life and a rock to me.

My dad, too, came to see the boys. He was so thrilled with them. It was a very special moment for him, for all of us, and for the first time we all felt like a family.

Tina visited with her children too. Her kids were all so lovely with the boys – she and I had taken a photo together in our last weeks of pregnancy and now we took another picture, in the same pose, holding the boys. I think this was probably the happiest time of my life and I feel so incredibly blessed to have been able to experience it.

My manager recommended I do one interview as my house was being watched by the paparazzi for a month for a valuable first picture of my boys. It drove me crazy so Vickie said, 'Well, if you give the pics to OK! magazine then the paps will go away as the pictures would be out. It sounded sensible and I trust her implicitly so I agreed to do it.

The day came for the *Daily Mail* journalist Jan Moir to do the interview and I was actually quite nervous. Not like me at all but I felt I'd been cocooned away from everything for weeks and now, here I was, plunging straight back in the deep end by talking to the *Mail*. Jan was great though and seemed very taken with the boys. I wasn't worried about my weight for these pictures. I'd probably lost about 20lbs by the time this interview came out in October, but I wasn't going to go into some sort of tailspin over my appearance. I was losing weight gradually because the boys were breastfeeding constantly and it felt as though I couldn't eat enough to keep up with them!

Having my hair and make-up done for the shoot was a luxury, though. I tried to kick back and enjoy that day, although I did forget to get my nails done! Disaster! I go from being a woman having a regular manicure, pedicure and weekly massages to a mom of two with chipped and raggedy nails, all in the space of a few weeks. But you know what? It was something of a relief, to just let go for a while and not have beauty treatments on my priority lists.

When the interview came out in the UK, again, I waited with baited breath to read those vile remarks people feel compelled to write under the *Mail Online* stories. But it wasn't as bad as I'd feared. There seemed to be genuine interest in my story. Mainly, people were completely obsessed about which baby was born to my carrier and which I gave birth to, but we decided to keep this information strictly between us as a family.

I want to protect the boys as much as I can and I certainly don't want them to feel any differently about themselves or about their parents because one of them was born to a carrier. I actually feel that I'm protecting the boys by sharing this story this way, no one can get it wrong – like the person who wrote a story saying I was adopting one of my children and neither of them were actually mine!

Both boys are biologically mine and Ty's; one of them just had a babysitter for nine months, to borrow Tina's phrase. And that's what we'll explain to the boys later, when they're older and when they're ready.

Of course, the next hoop we needed to jump through was making sure we could bring our boys back to the UK.

I felt I couldn't relax at all until all the papers were in order. There's a constant, niggling fear that something could go wrong, and it persisted right up until the time we were rubber stamped and were able to bring the boys home without any worries.

It is sadly much, much harder to use a surrogate in the UK than in the US because the British legal system doesn't seem to want to encourage surrogacy in any way, even though, clearly, it's going on all the time. It seems very unfair really, when there are desperate parents and women happy to be carriers, but the fact is, there's a real suspicion around the procedure over here.

The way it stands in the UK now is that surrogacy arrangements are unenforceable by UK law, although in fact, there have only been two UK cases in the last ten years or so where surrogates have refused to give up the baby, and that's out of almost 1000 births, so it's pretty unlikely this would happen to you if you were considering surrogacy. But even so, no one wants to have any risk involved with having your biological child taken from you and having the right to do so.

If you're interested in looking into surrogacy, remember every country has different laws and you'll need to employ the best legal help you can afford in order to guarantee your child can't be taken from you and to guarantee your carrier has no legal recourse at the end of the process. I researched long and hard to find the best agency and legal advice. They are highly reputable and they offered so much support and guidance for the carrier and parents. Don't expect this as a given; a lot of agencies don't offer this.

An organisation called Brilliant Beginnings is trying to change the law here in the UK and are also experts in surrogacy and egg donation. The details are at the back of this book but their campaigning lawyer, Natalie Gamble, is leading the campaign for legal changes on surrogacy in the UK. Worth looking her up if you're in need of advice on this.

Right after my children were born we had to submit their birth certificates to get their passports. To get a birth certificate in the US can take up to six months and we wanted to go home right away. We had no idea how long this process was going to take.

I stalked the officials at the town hall every single day, driving 45 minutes each way. I think they just got sick of me and that's why they processed the birth certificates so quickly.

And then we had to submit the birth certificates so they could get their passports. In this case there was no one to stalk so we just had to sit tight. We were so lucky; they came through within a couple of weeks and there were no complications in terms of the surrogacy: I was their mom and Ty was their dad.

We finally made it home to the UK in October 2013 and I'll never forget stepping over the threshold into our new home. This was our new life with our boys and it was just beginning. I couldn't wait to introduce them to friends and family – they already had their names down for nursery school and pre-prep.

It was such a relief to walk through the door of our new home, put the kettle on and make a proper cup of green tea. That's one way in which I'm not an honorary Brit! On top of that, I'd still say that my ambition and how I express it is very American. Speaking of which, for obvious reasons, my business had very much taken a back seat. For a few months at least there was not one iota of me thinking about work – it was all about my children. All I wanted to do was to be with my boys.

It's strange: I didn't ever consider moving to the States after the boys were born. I've been here in the UK for so long, as has Ty, that I can't imagine living anywhere else. As the boys grow up, they'll have English accents and their parents will speak with an American twang! Funny that I've ended up with an American guy too, when so many boyfriends were Brits. Maybe there's some deep-seated affinity we have with each other because we're from Stateside. Or maybe it's because Ty is just so damn hot!

Chapter 17

The Next Chapter

No matter how wrapped up in babyworld I was, on landing back in the UK I had my work cut out. The October By Caprice campaign went down fantastically well and sold in huge numbers: Lucy Meck (as she's known) was perfect for us. But I had to push on. The business had been my baby for so long and I'd been neglecting it. During IVF, pregnancy and the birth I'd taken my eye off the ball and I needed to be there for my team because without a team leader, with all the best intentions, the direction of the company can drift a little. I needed to focus, at the same time as getting used to this whole new world of being mommy to my boys.

Retail is incredibly tough – way more than it ever has been – and I doubt I could do it again if I was starting from scratch today – but I have a brand, which is so important in the marketplace, and whilst By Caprice is a relatively small brand, I do have big plans in the pipeline.

I don't know why people are always surprised at how involved I am with my business and the knowledge I have of it. For goodness' sake, I don't have any equity partners, I have always owned 100 per cent of my business. In the beginning I put in a little over £250,000 to open up the doors and I continued to invest capital for the first two years. At that point, I started to make my money back. In any small business they say it usually takes around three years to make your investment back.

I've always had to fight for everything I have in my life and I've always had a very ambitious work ethic.

I do a lot of seminars and corporate speeches in front of fellow business owners and entrepreneurs who are starting out, and students. After all, they are our future. I love doing this, by the way; I meet people whom I learn a lot from and I love to inspire people and share my lessons and tools on how to start a small business and succeed in this economy. I always tell people: know every integral part of your business, have passion for what you do, live it and breathe it and have pride in your product, as customers aren't impulsive like they used to be. They want quality and a good price and if you don't give it to them, a competitor will. Cash flow is your bible – you have to know what's going in and going out for the next nine months. If there's a problem, you have the time to find solutions now. Don't be greedy, look after your team and they will look after you. Be agile in business, use and invest in social media... I could go on and on about this but it would be an entirely different book.

Anyway, back to my boys.

When they were six months old I went back to work: I'd

dipped in and out in between the office and home but the business needed more of my attention now. The way I do things has had to change, of course; I'm finding the guilt pretty hard to deal with sometimes because being at work means being away from the boys. But I remember that I didn't miss my mom when she was at work because we had our housekeeper Lupé to look after us and we had lots of family nearby. We were really happy kids and my mom was happy because she was doing something she loved; I draw inspiration from that.

I have changed in that I never go away for more than a couple of days at a stretch. I used to go away for weeks at a time but now, if I have to go to my factories in China, to spec in my new collection and source materials, I'll constantly be Facetiming the boys. Last time I was there I'd tell the people in the meeting I needed to go to the loo and I'd disappear for ages to call them. It was embarrassing as they kept asking if my stomach was OK.

I miss the boys so much, whether I'm in a meeting or away, but I'm hoping this will pass. Mom tells me it gets easier and I guess we just get used to it as time goes by and the children become more independent. Whenever I do my business speeches I just tell people we have to do the best we can – and I really do believe that it's different for working women. Men just don't seem to feel guilty. I think they'd feel guilty if they couldn't support their child, but for women it's a more complex emotional thing.

My business is expanding and I'm in talks to create new ranges and branch out in all kinds of exciting ways. Motherhood has also made me more creative and opened my eyes to new opportunities. It's enriched me and brought a burning fire. I'm smarter and even more ambitious.

And there's something else – something important that has come out of my journey to become a mom. I'm determined to help other women by talking openly about IVF and infertility. Now that women know I've had IVF I've discovered how many of them out there are desperate for a child or have had problems with conceiving.

It's a visceral pain that women feel – like an open wound. I know that it's incredibly hard for men, too, especially when they see the woman they love going through this physically difficult, emotionally scarring time of their lives but I wonder if it's as damaging to a man's self-esteem as it seems to be for some women.

Personally, I know that if I'd not managed to have a child, I'd have spiralled down into the depths of despair, because there's something so fundamental about wanting to hold your child, nurture them, see them grow and know that you've helped to create this person. It's almost primal and with all the pain and anxiety I went through, it really, really made me appreciate the experiences of other women. Getting yourself up and running again, dusting yourself off and moving on takes time and it takes effort. I always think it's a grieving process and with all grief, I think you have to just take it a day at time and not expect too much.

That said, if I'd not been able to have children, I hope I would have found a way forward somehow, as so many women do. I'm not sure how, or what I'd have done because it would have meant totally adjusting my dreams for the future, but us girls are good at improvising and we find ways to nurture in different ways.

I'm not sure if this is age or if it's becoming a mother (or both) but I find it increasingly difficult to stay emotionally detached whenever I'm confronted by women with sick children or single moms who are struggling hard to bring up their kids because of finances or otherwise.

Ty and I attend balls and various charity events throughout the year and they're often fun but all with deeply moving stories behind them. In the past I raised about a quarter of a million pounds hosting a ball to raise money for Childline, which was just great – and I helped raise quite a lot of money for Great Ormond Street Hospital.

But sometimes it's just about receiving a tweet from someone who's having a terrible time with their child, which happened only the other night when someone sent me a photo of their little girl. The child couldn't eat and she had tubes coming out of her nose; of course I broke down (and I wouldn't have done a few years ago – the boys opened the floodgates!) and sent some money to the foundation her parents had set up to help cure her. How could I not, when I have the money to give?

I'm so grateful for everything I have and I think it's so important to think about other people who don't have it so good. If you do work hard and make a lot of money, then you should be giving back too. It doesn't matter what you give: 1 per cent, 5 per cent or 10 per cent – just give. If you've earned your money it also puts you in a position of responsibility. God dang it, we have to help make a positive change in the world.

Even when I was a young girl of 16, three times a week I would drive myself and donate my time working with the mentally disabled. I would also send money to various charities; it wasn't much, only a few dollars a month but if I could make a change in even one person's life then it was worth the effort.

I support quite a few charities and help out where I can but it's very hard because each cause is worthwhile in different ways and you can't support everything.

I was introduced to the Woman's Trust, which is a charity working across London, by a lady I knew through my local taxi company. She always answered the phone and I'd book cars through her all the time. One day we had a little talk and she told me about the fact that she'd had a terrible time as a victim of domestic violence. She explained that a tiny charity called Woman's Trust had helped her to get away and now she volunteers for them but they were really struggling with funding: they were about to lose all the money from the government that helped them to provide counsellors for these women.

I wanted to find out more and I went to meet some of their clients – the ladies who were using the charity's services – and to hear about their experiences. I won't go into any detail but one had ended up living in a refuge for a while to escape her abusive partner, and another woman had been through such a long, sustained period of abuse she'd lost all her confidence and until she discovered the Woman's Trust, she'd felt completely trapped by her circumstances.

What I've realised over the years is that abuse comes in all shapes and sizes and doesn't just happen to the under-privileged. I've had friends who have – for whatever reasons – been dependent on their partners, I think because the men wanted it that way, to retain control. These women have ended up with no power or influence and with an abusive partner they feel unable to escape. These men make them feel inadequate, they tell them they'll never find another man and that they can't survive on their own and as a result, these women feel dependent and they end up accepting the abuse. We've got to help change this.

I have a very beautiful friend who used to have her own business. She was very successful and when she got together with this man, he serially undermined her until over time she lost all her confidence. Now he'll say to her, 'Nobody looks at you, you're so ugly,' but really, he's doing this because he has no confidence of his own and it's the only way he thinks he can keep this girl ... He's a pig, he looks like one and acts like one.

Over time she's become a ghost of the girl she used to be. The verbal abuse is shocking and she honestly feels she has nowhere to go and no one to turn to because he controls everything. A charity like Woman's Trust is there to help out women like this, to provide one-to-one counselling for women who feel they've reached the end of their tether and just don't know where to go for help. This is to plug that gap.

For me, hearing what these women had to say, I knew I had to help. The charity was within weeks of closing down because they had no money and yet in Westminster alone, the borough I live in, there were over 1300 cases of domestic violence in 2014. Needless to say, the services in Westminster did not close.

Until I began looking into this, I had no idea that domestic violence was so prevalent. It is so shocking: I found out that one in four women in the UK experience domestic violence at some point in their lives and that two women a week die as a result of a violent partner in the UK. That's outright murder, whichever way you look at it, and I was so shocked that this was happening on my doorstep. I wanted to help if at all possible.

And so that's what I did – I've become patron of the Woman's Trust and we have plans to put the spotlight on it as soon as possible. I've been supporting it for three years now. It's tiny but it's so important and they do wonderful work helping women regain their confidence and self-esteem. They are now able to fund 50 counsellors across London and it's a wonderful feeling to be able to help.

There are other charities I support too – one called Tikva, which helps orphans in the Ukraine. The charity is based in Odessa and you wouldn't believe the places they rescue the children from. Some of them are living in sewers or hovels, sleeping on floors. They have such desperate childhoods and this charity is helping them to have a home, food and education... a future. Ty and I have three children we fully support and they'll never have to go and live on the streets again. I am also working hard to create the awareness to raise funds so that other children will have this opportunity as well.

I've had to narrow down the charities I can work with and support and now I try to make them about women who are suffering abuse or about children, but even that covers so many different areas that it's hard to know where to stop. But still, it's a necessity and I want to step up to the challenge as often and whenever I can.

Chapter 18

Home is Where the Heart is

I'm not as famous as I used to be… and that's just fine by me. Honestly, my life now is about my children. It's not about me any more, it's about me and my family and my business: because By Caprice is going to give my kids a great future. It's a business I built all on my own without anyone else's financial backing and I'm really proud of it.

I will still do the TV appearances but I'll choose the projects very carefully, with my children in mind. I have a huge responsibility to them and to my stepchildren to make good decisions about the projects I do. So if *Strictly* came knocking, I'd do it (if the timing was right); shows I've done like *Who's Doing the Dishes* are just fun and light, or *Posh Pawn* – it was for charity and it was fun too, a double whammy! But really, the kind of work I do from now on has to be good and inspiring.

There are people who'll wonder why I've written this book. I know they'll say, 'It's too personal, why do you feel the need to capitalise on your life story?' But my answer is: it's a beautiful story. I didn't think I could have children yet somehow, we managed it. And by talking about miscarriage, surrogacy and the hardships people go through to have children, I really hope it breaks some taboos for people – and that people will celebrate my story with me – and most importantly I hope it will inspire many people not to give up hope on their dream of becoming parents.

I've made plenty of mistakes across the years but I want to do things the right way now, in a way that makes my family proud of me.

Last night I was sitting at home, the kids tucked up in bed and Ty away on business. I sat there texting six of my girlfriends, catching up with them, finding out how they're doing and I caught myself thinking, who'd ever have thought I'd be such a girlie girl?

These days I have virtually no male friends at all and I seem to have lost the ability to flirt. When I look back to the years in my twenties and thirties with all the parties and the men and the crazy travel, I feel a little nostalgic but I don't miss it at all. You couldn't pay me £10m to go back to that period of my life. I had a wild time and I loved it, wouldn't swap it for anything. But now I have everything I could ever want or need in this one place. Me and my boys: my family is everything.

When I met Ty, I discovered a side to myself I'd never experienced before, a nurturing side that wanted to explore the side of life money just can't buy. I lost my ambition, temporarily at least – but that drive came out in other ways, in the way I felt this huge unconditional love for someone else I really wanted to have a family with. And all the men I'd met before or had relationships with before paled into insignificance when I met Ty; they were there to help me appreciate this Prince Charming who eventually came into my life.

Ty and I are like high schoolers, we'll just sit in bed eating popcorn and goofing around. I'll tell him he's gorgeous and he tells me off for being so soppy. He's 150 per cent my soul mate and I'm more in love with him now than ever before and I love hanging out with him because he's my best friend – and of course I want to tear his clothes off every five minutes.

It's not easy though, this constant juggle and the switch between roles, as every working woman with children knows. It's tough because we have to be Wonder Woman, don't we: we have to work and look after the children and look after our man. I cannot stress this enough: men and women are fundamentally so different and women just have to be multi-taskers.

It's not like the old days when the men were just going out to earn the money whilst the women stayed home. It's too expensive these days and anyway, I for one wouldn't want to be a woman who had no earning power of her own.

It's kind of empowering to know that you, too, are a bread-winner of the family but also, the whole foundation of the family is down to us women; we're the glue that holds it all together and the inspiration for our kids.

I've seen family relationships shifting and changing since the children have come along. Ty's children love the boys to pieces and they're so wonderful together when they're all with us. I love having a houseful; I'm forever saying, 'Come on over, bring your friends, bring your whole class if you want!' because I grew up with so much family around me and I love that feeling of coming full-circle.

Ty's dad, Bill, is an incredible person who has become a fatherly figure in my life and has been instrumental in getting my dad and me in touch again. Bill is one of the smartest human beings: he's dynamic and quite intimidating! He has the ability to see straight through anyone in seconds, he'll clock you and know exactly what you're about. He's a wonderful man and Ty has lots of his qualities.

When I say to Ty, 'You're so kind, you're so good, honey,' he gets so mad!

'Why can't you say I'm really hot or something?' he'll grin at me. But he has kindness and integrity in spades. And there's not many people around with real integrity these days, I can tell you.

I'm glad that Dad has seen the boys and that Bill pushed me a little to reach out to my father. I don't want my dad to have any headaches; I want my dad to be happy and if he wants to see me he knows my number. There's no animosity between us, there's only love from me – and I have to believe he feels the same way. He's pushing 70 now and he's not very well. I wish him only the best.

As far as my mom goes, I'm just so grateful to her for everything she's done for me, the way she brought me up and the way she loves my boys so much. These days, it's all about the boys for her, she's not that interested in me and that's the way it should be! It's all about nurturing the next generation.

My mom and I have both softened with age. I never thought I could learn to be so empathetic and patient but it's happened since I had the boys and my mom loves it! She's become much more vulnerable and emotional, maybe because I've softened towards her or maybe it's just age!

So the wild child has become a bit more earth mother – but still with the same drive and ambition I've always had, just firing off in new directions now. I waited 39 years to meet the right man. I had a tough time having my children and now the next step on this journey is to make sure my family are brought up with good, old-fashioned values of respect, hard work and a big, squishy hug from their mom whenever they need it. I don't know what the next chapter of my life holds but I'm glad I have Ty, my kids and his to share it with.